HELP ME SAY IT

HELP ME SAY IT

A Parent's Guide to Speech Problems

By CAROL BARACH

1817

HARPER & ROW, PUBLISHERS, New York

Cambridge, Philadelphia, San Francisco, London
Mexico City, São Paulo, Sydney

FIRST EDITION

Designer: Sidney Feinberg

Library of Congress Cataloging in Publication Data

Barach, Carol.
  Help me say it.

  Bibliography: p.
  Includes index.
  1. Speech disorders in children.   2. Speech therapy for children.   I. Title.
RJ496.S7B36   1983   618.92′855   83–47525
ISBN 0–06–181046–0

---

83 84 85 86 87 10 9 8 7 6 5 4 3 2 1

To Andrea, David and the memory of Lex

Contents

Acknowledgments

Many people have helped on this book, and I am grateful to all of them. Dr. Freeman McConnell, my professor as a graduate student, gave me help and support on the hearing chapter. Zenobia Bagli also helped straighten me out on hearing disorders. Jill Copeland of the Association of Retarded Citizens of Davidson County, Tennessee, was a valuable resource. She put me in touch with some parents of handicapped students who shared their experiences with me. Susie Baird, Margaret Allison and Pat Butler taught me that raising a handicapped child can have positive effects rather than be an experience of nothing but grief and discouragement. These women show how such a challenge can be met creatively and successfully. I must also thank my mother, Caroline Bird, who felt I should write this book and even thought that I could. I would also like to mention my stepfather, the late Tom Mahoney, whose support and practical advice early in this project were very helpful. My husband, John Paul Barach, has lived and suffered through all the stages of this project and deserves some acknowledgment for endurance and patience. He also willingly did some calculations that only a physicist could do. My daughter Andrea Schine must be mentioned, as she is the person who led me into this profession in the first place. My son, David, was my laboratory in child and language development. Jerry Gross must be credited with the idea for this book in the first place. He has edited many versions of the book with patience and diligence and has managed to clean up my tangled prose to make it readable. Carol Cohen gave this book the focus and shape it has. Her editing has not only enabled me to communicate to the reader in a useful way but taught me how to write a book.

Foreword

This book was written for parents whose children have some kind of communication problem or fear that there might be one. Of all the handicaps I can think of, from blindness to paralysis, the inability to talk to other people seems the most devastating, for without communication each of us is completely alone. The only way we can know what goes on in other people's minds is through the communication system we know as language, either spoken or written. If this communication system is impaired at any point— sending, receiving, comprehending—we cannot take our place in our culture or society.

Parenting is an activity done mostly by talking and listening. Not only would we be concerned if our children suffered impaired communication, but we would also be handicapped in our efforts to rear such a child. We would have to learn *some* manner of communication to serve as a bridge between our child and the rest of the world. To some extent all parents do this, but those with a disabled child must do it better and longer.

Bringing up children is not easy, even under the best conditions, but a child with problems, severe or mild, offers an extra challenge. No one is properly trained for parenthood, but other parents can share their experiences with us. When our child has a special problem, though, we are on our own.

Today's parents do not have the support system enjoyed by earlier generations. Young couples often have their first baby far from their own parents, in a new town where they do not even have many friends. They may have come from small families themselves and have had no real experience with small children until they have the complete responsibility for their own. It is not surprising then that they do not know what to expect. They cannot tell if their child is developing normally, because they have no knowledge of what a normal child does as a comparison. The usual professional advice received by parents is from physicians who are mainly concerned with the physical well-being of children. They are not prepared to give parents the kind of guidance they need in helping their children in other areas of development.

I know this because I was there myself. My first child talked strangely (to my ears) when she was four and five years old. Luckily we lived quite near the Bill Wilkerson Hearing and Speech Center. There was a big design of an ear and a mouth on the door, and I thought that this might be the right place to go. So, never having heard of speech therapy, we went in. The articulation problem cleared up easily. My child was dismissed from therapy, but I stayed on as a student. I had never thought of speech one way or the other, having always been able to say whatever I had wanted to. But when I was forced to think about it, I realized that it was a truly remarkable ability which would be considered astonishing were it not so commonplace. Now every time I talk to a parent, I remember when I was a parent talking to the speech clinician.

Over the years, my clinical experience has taught me that the most crucial factor in the outcome of speech therapy is parental support and effort. As I look over the chapters of this book I find I emphasize this again and again. I have seen a tendency for parents to leave it to the experts to solve their problems. They feel that they are powerless to take action themselves. I must admit that this attitude is often encouraged by some of my colleagues who give parents the impression that they are more hindrance than help. Many professionals are threatened by the "overaggressive" mother or father. But the children of these "overaggressive" parents do better! It is up to the professional to guide and teach the parents so that they can teach their children. There are not enough clinicians in the world nor is there money enough to pay them (no matter how wealthy the parents might be), to have all speech hearing and language therapy professionally handled. The bulk of the burden falls where it has always fallen—on the parents.

Another factor in the probability of therapy success is how early treatment is started. I emphasize throughout the book the need to get help as soon as possible. Time, the crucial factor in child development, passes more quickly than parents realize. Six months in a toddler's life is a large proportion of the child's whole existence. Generally speaking, the earliest intervention possible is best for a child with a communication problem. Of course if all problems are treated as early as possible there will inevitably be some which would have cleared up on their own. Therefore from the point of view of the professional or the school there is a tendency to see if children can "grow" out of the difficulty in order to use funds and resources most efficiently. As a parent, however, you are not interested in the efficiency of resource use, you are interested in giving your child the best possible chance. Parents not only must look at their child objectively but must uncover the resources available for their child in the community. This book has been written with these attitudes in mind.

This book also is for the parent who first discovers a communication problem. Professional expertise is not needed to identify or diagnose the problem. The parent does need to recognize the possible presence of a problem and seek help if there is a question about the child's communicative ability. It is hoped that this book will not only answer questions parents may have on the various types of communication problems, but help them to find services and understand what can be expected from these services. In addition I hope this book will also aid parents to understand how to manage their children within the family group to help them overcome a communication difficulty.

The first chapter outlines normal speech and language development. It contains the information I wish I had had when I first watched a baby learn to talk. The second chapter gives the various types of communication disorders in children. This chapter also contains the normal timetable of development as well as warning signals for parents which may indicate communication problems as early as possible. The next six chapters treat the various disorders—how a parent can identify them, how to get help and what the parent can do at home to remedy the difficulty. The last chapter is a resource chapter which tells about the types of speech and hearing services available, how to find them and what to expect from them. There is an appendix at the end of the book which gives various organizations—with addresses and telephone numbers (when possible) that parents can use to obtain further information. There is also a recommended reading list for more information on specific aspects of communication disorders. Footnotes give some specific sources and elaboration on some points in the text.

What do you call a speech and hearing professional? This book uses several terms: speech clinician, speech teacher, speech pathologist, speech/language pathologist. What is the difference? Very little except the name. The person who helps others speak is called by different names in different places. We used to be known as *speech correctionists*. Many did not like the name because it had an authoritarian ring to it and did not suggest a helping profession. Then we were called speech therapists and the people we helped were called patients. I feel this has a cozy and warm connotation and personally would have been happy to remain a speech therapist. Unfortunately the term *therapist* has some legal implications, referring as it does to a person who works under a medical doctor's supervision. The term had to be dropped so that we could maintain our professional independence. The term *speech pathologist* came into use and the subject was called speech pathology. Although the word *pathology* simply means disease or disorder, I have been unhappy with the term being used for our profession because it is often confused with a medical pathologist whose subjects most certainly do not have speech problems. But it sticks, with the addition of *language* (as in *speech/language pathologist*) as the official term according to the American Speech-Language-Hearing Association (also known as ASHA). Since that is such a mouthful to say, I often use the term *speech clinician*, which is accurate. In the United Kingdom, and many of the English-speaking countries outside the United States, the term *speech therapist* is often used as the official name.

The children in this book, although they are based upon my experiences with real children, are composites of several children I have known. But none of them is an actual person. There might be some similarity to real children, but that is as it should be because they are used to illustrate real problems and real situations. In actual clinic practice it would be unusual to have such clear-cut cases that described a disorder so precisely.

I hope that my fictional children will help you identify your own child's difficulties and my fictional parents can serve as guides for your actions and attitudes in the help you give your own children.

Parents are not the only ones who can help children in trouble; other members of the family can also aid in the effort to teach a child to communicate. Grandparents, uncles, aunts, brothers and sisters can have important roles in the child's communication environment. Parents who have an extended family nearby are very fortunate. The child who relates or has access to many people in day-to-day social interchange has an advantage. If your situation is not so lucky, find and join a parents' group no matter what your professional treatment program is. Not only do you have a lot to learn from other parents, you have a lot to teach them. As parents you have special knowledge and insight that no professional can have. Whether or not you are an expert in speech, hearing or language, you are the expert in your child.

1

Your Baby Learns to Talk

- *The First Six Months*
- *The Second Six Months*
- *One Year Old*
- *Two and Three Years*
- *Four to Six Years*
- *As Your Child Learns to Speak: Suggestions for Parents*

The First Six Months

Little Sarah is finally home. The long wait is over, the admiring relatives have all gone, and you are alone with your new baby. She is lying in her bassinet, and you know you've never before seen such perfection. But when she looks at you, what is she thinking? You don't know because she can't tell you. But you do know that in a few short years she *will* talk. Is it your responsibility to teach her? How *can* you teach your baby to talk? Suppose you don't do it right? Being responsible for another human being is wonderful but also frightening, and you feel poorly prepared for the awesome task. How can you let Sarah know how much you love her? How can you communicate with her? Suddenly her face screws up, her little mouth opens wide, and she cries. She has just communicated with you. Forgetting your apprehensive thoughts about parenthood, you pick her up, decide she is hungry and feed her. You have communicated with her by providing the milk she drinks and holding her in your arms. You and Sarah have set up your first communication system.

Learning to Talk Starts at Birth

You may not realize it, but Sarah has already started to learn to talk. She began in her first few minutes of life when she took her first breath and breathed out while crying. (When you speak you coordinate your breathing out with running your voice box. Exhaled breath is the power behind talking.) The first thing Sarah did in this world was to put together breathing and vocalization. She has already started to vocalize, a skill necessary for talking, and to communicate, the reason for talking. Long before she says her first word, she will be building her language. You do not have to teach her how to learn a language. Nature has provided her with the capacity to pick up a language without any special instruction.[1] But you do have to provide her with the raw material of the particular language of your culture and with the psychological environment that enhances her natural ability to learn to talk. Her natural capacity will never be realized without you. You may not know consciously *how* you talk, but you do know how *to* talk, and that is enough to give Sarah the example or speech model she needs.

Even before Sarah was born she lived in a sound environment. Her mother's womb was fairly noisy, always full of gurgles and rumblings and heartbeats. (Many babies seem to like repetitive sounds like a ticking clock—perhaps they miss their mother's heartbeat.) The first time Sarah heard silence was probably *after* she was born. Sarah's new world, however, is full of many kinds of sensation. She sees constantly shifting lights and shapes, but it will take some time before she can make sense out of them. She hears many new sounds, most of which don't make sense yet. The sensation which does have immediate meaning for Sarah is her sense of touch. When you hold her she feels safe and secure. She enjoys nursing, and her mouth is the part of her body of which Sarah is most aware. Her mouth is the place of her greatest enjoyment and also the means of communication with those who care for her. When something is not perfect in Sarah's world she cries. Not only

1. Modern linguistic theory as developed by Eric Lenneberg and Noam Chomsky and others is that language is part of the biological heritage of the human being. We are born with a mental organization of grammar and need to learn the specific words in order to use it. This can be compared to a computer wired for various logical operations which needs a program to use them.

are her simple needs communicated in this way but the cries also provide practice in working the voice, lips, tongue, jaw and lungs together, a necessity for talking.

Practicing New Sounds

A baby's cries change almost daily. Sarah's crying starts out in the first week as a series of open-mouth cries of the same loudness sounding like the *a* in *hat*. In two weeks her cries change from monotonous repetitions to ones with real expression. The pitch and volume both vary (from a whimper to a shriek) and the cries are either long or short. At one month Sarah adds some new sounds to her repertoire: llllllll, rrrrrrrr, guh, mmmmmmmm, sucking sounds, lip and tongue smacking sounds. She begins to make sounds for the fun of it instead of only crying to complain about some need that was not being met. Sarah's playing with her mouth and experimenting with its movements is good for her. While awake she explores the inside of her mouth, more concerned with the feelings of her movements than with the sounds she produces with them.

If you listen to Sarah very carefully in that period between two and six months you may be surprised to hear all kinds of sounds. Some sounds will be like those you use in English but there will be others which are definitely foreign: the *ch* of German, the Spanish *r* and some you may not be able to identify. You may be puzzled because you know that Sarah has not heard such sounds. You may also remember how hard it was to learn to say some of these sounds when you studied a foreign language in school. Since deaf children also experiment with their mouths at this stage and seem to produce many different speech sounds, speech pathologists believe that babies at this stage are not listening to the sounds but rather playing with the movements. Sarah is not really trying to make sounds during this first half year, but attempting all the possible movements with her mouth. Her enormous repertoire of sounds tells you that they are the result of experimentation rather than the attempt to reproduce specific language sounds she has heard. If you think about how *you* talk, you realize that the feel of making the words is a large part of how you know you are talking and how you know what you are saying. You are now very used to how it feels to talk but you started learning this feeling when you were only a month old. At this beginning stage, Sarah does not know whether someday she will be speaking Japanese, Arabic, Polish or whatever and practices all the movements for the sounds just in case. When she is older and uses only the English sounds she hears, all the non-English sounds will disappear from lack of practice.

Communication Skills Increase

You will notice that Sarah is communicating better and that you can understand more easily her wants and needs by her cries. She has probably trained you to understand her needs at the same time the sounds of her cries have changed. These cries have different meanings, depending on what is wrong. At six to eight weeks, however, you start a two-way communication. When Sarah smiles, you're delighted and return the smile. This communication is complete, and one that is unique to human beings. Sarah's response to your smile means that she must be aware not only of faces but what facial expressions say. She also understands the emotional content of talk by listening to the tone of your voice. It is not too early to help your baby associate talking with pleasure. When you hold Sarah and talk to her in a warm and loving way, she will connect the sound of your voice with something she enjoys doing. In these early months, it doesn't matter so much *what* you say but *how* you say it. Some people believe that babies are sensitive to the emotional message in speech because they are not distracted by the sense of words. Most parents realize that the tone of their voice is very important in talking with a baby and so they tend to exaggerate their vocal expressions. They also tend to exaggerate their facial expressions. Avoid the overdone tone of voice which often becomes sing-song and too extreme smiles, frowns, etc. Strive for more natural behavior, one that will be consistent, making it easier for Sarah to read people's faces and understand their tones of voice. Get into the habit of using the same words with the same gestures, and Sarah's future understanding of words will be helped by her early comprehension of tone of voice and gesture.[2]

2. L. Bloom and M. Lahey, *Language Development and Language Disorders* (New York: John Wiley and Sons, 1978). The communicative value of speech comes earlier in life than we used to think, according to recent research. Newborn babies' movements can be seen to be synchronized with the adult speech they hear. Vocalization in three-month-old infants changes in kind and amount in different physical situations and in response to adult speech. Therefore the baby seems to be responsive to the speech environment from a very early age.

Sarah has been aware of speech from others. Now, at five months, she turns toward the sound of the person talking. She stares at the mouths of people as they talk, recognizing not only speech but the exact place from which it comes. You have been talking to her all along as you care for her, and so she has learned that talk is a social activity long before she knows the meanings of the words.

It is important in these first six months not only to provide Sarah with social stimulation but to allow her some time on her own to pursue the exploration of her mouth. You may have noticed that when you appear as she is experimenting with her mouth, she stops and pays attention to you. It is important that she know her mouth completely to prepare for the difficult task of forming the speech sounds to say words.

Do not be concerned during the first six months that Sarah does not make any attempt to imitate you. It may be too difficult for her now. Before Sarah imitates you, you might try to demonstrate imitation by imitating *her*. If she bangs her toy on the floor, you bang it the same way. If Sarah says *bah* you say *bah*. This game is usually a big hit with babies. When Sarah becomes able to imitate you, she will turn the game around herself.

Listening to and Imitating Herself

Around five or six months you may notice a change in Sarah's vocal experimentation: sounds are repeated. Instead of *ba* you hear *ba ba* or even *ba ba ba ba ba ba ba*. Not only is Sarah practicing the feeling of saying *ba*, she is listening to the result of her experiment.[3] She repeats it to make it last longer. She is also imitating the sound she hears herself making. This is the start of the feedback pattern that Sarah and the rest of us use all our lives. What we say is heard not only by the listener but by ourselves; we judge how it sounds, and modify our speech production if necessary so that the result is precisely what we want. Sarah will find this procedure necessary as she learns to say words. She hears the word you say, listens to her own attempt, judges it and modifies it to make her pronunciation as perfect as possible. When Sarah begins to listen to herself she also begins listening more closely to others. Now the imitation game can be played both ways. Since you supply her

3. There is some evidence that deaf babies do not repeat syllables, indicating that the ability to hear is the reason for the repetitions.

with English sounds, you shape her sound repertoire. The foreign sounds disappear, leaving only the English sounds for her to practice. She also imitates your tone of voice.

The Second Six Months

Putting Words to Things and Events

In her second half year, when she begins to crawl and later to walk, Sarah may abandon her speechlike activities for a while. She is too busy exploring the physical world. Help her by making that world stimulating, full of textures, colors and sounds. She needs some time to explore these things alone, but at other times you can talk about them with her and provide her with the words with which to think about them. You may be surprised to find that Sarah understands some words long before she says them. Supply her with words to go along with what she is doing, "Roll the ball," "Put the ball in the box," "Squeeze the ball," etc. You are not telling her what to do, you are merely describing what she is already doing. Accompany your own activities with words. "Wash the dish. Dry the dish. Put the dish away." Thus Sarah experiences the real world and the auditory symbols (words) for the real world at the same time. This connection will be clearer to Sarah if you can keep the sentences short and the words simple. Center your talk on the here and now. Something that is going to happen in the future won't have much meaning for her. Something that happened an hour ago is ancient history and not interesting to her. Sarah is, however, beginning to recognize a predictable sequence of routine. She may understand that after supper comes bathtime and after her bathtime comes bedtime. Such routine is important for babies; it makes them feel secure and also helps in their understanding of the organization of the real world. The pairing of the words to the events is another routine and predictable procedure. Sarah has a lot to learn: cups of liquid with steam rising from them can hurt her; the shiny red apple tastes sweet and nice but the shiny red ball tastes awful. If you supply Sarah with the words, she will not only learn the words but will better understand the events they relate to. Drink some milk, All gone. No no. Come here. Blow your nose. Peek-a-boo. Fall down. Sarah understands sentences such as these at about ten months. You know she understands because her response is accurate. Now, not only is she reading expression and gesture but she is picking out the meaning of what you say by the sounds of the words themselves.

Picking Out Meaning from a Torrent of Speech Sounds

Learning to understand words is a mighty task, one you have done for so long that you take it for granted. But you can experience the difficulty of it somewhat if you have had the experience of being in a foreign country that uses a language you have never heard. Not only don't you know what the words mean, you can't even tell when one word ends and the next begins. You can't even pick out the sounds that make the words because you don't know what to listen for. You know that in English the *p* in *pill* is the same sound as the *p* in *lip* even though they are different. One is aspirated, the other is not. You can tell the *p* in *pill* is aspirated if you put your hand near your mouth while saying *pill*. You will feel a puff of air. When you put your hand near your mouth and say *lip* you will not feel the puff of air from the unaspirated *p*. This difference makes no difference to you and you hear the two sounds as the same basic sound. In another language, however, this difference between the aspirated *p* (with the puff of air) and the unaspirated *p* (without the puff) is as great as the difference between *p* and *b* is for you as in the difference between *pill* and *bill*. Furthermore, there are some sounds you can't identify and never do hear accurately.

Sarah is learning to listen for the differences that change the meanings of words (such as the *p* and *b* in *pill* and *bill*) but to ignore those differences in the speech of those she listens to which do not change the meaning of words. She has not only to sort out all these speech sounds which come in at lightning speed, but to generalize that the word *cookie* said by Mama and the word *cookie* said by Daddy stand for the same thing, although the sound sensation is quite different in pitch and quality. Therefore Sarah must listen to the components of the word *cookie* said by Mama and by Daddy that are shared by both in order to understand the word. One of the major hurdles Sarah has in learning the way words sound and ascribing meaning to them is that they are over so fast. You can help by prolonging your words a bit to give Sarah extra time to take in the sound. You can also repeat the word or say it several times.

One Year Old

The Baby's First Word

At about a year you will be expecting your baby to say a real meaningful word. You will be playing out a drama that has been performed many times in the course of human history; nevertheless, it is always a hit.

Sarah is in her crib enthralled as usual with the sound of her own voice. You, her parents, are in the next room. Sarah says *mmmmm* and adds a vowel *mmma mmma*. You hear and run to Sarah. Sarah says, "Mma ma." Your face is all smiles as you pick up the baby, hug her and exclaim, "'Mama.' You said your first word, 'mama'!" Sarah says, "Mmmma ma mmmma ma." This is a wonderful word. You put Sarah down and start to go to the other room, but Sarah says "Mmma ma." This is *really* a magic word. It not only starts mother hugging her and making a delightful fuss over her but brings her from another room. This is not only fun, it is power. Thus Mommy has been named by baby. Sarah may not have meant to say her first meaningful word at that time, but Mommy supplied the meaning. Sarah found that *ma ma* didn't have the same magic with the other parent and it wasn't until she stumbled upon *da da* that Daddy got as excited as Mommy with *ma ma*. If you look at the baby names for mother and father in most languages, they are made up from baby double syllables that are easy for beginning speakers to say. Thus when the Italian baby accidentally hits on "ba bo" (Babbo), the Italian father knows that the baby has named him. All words are not learned in this accidental way, but it may be that Sarah learns that she can say words from this group of sounds.

Sarah's first couple of words were such a success that she branches out from there. She discovers that words not only communicate precisely what she wants to say but they are magic, they make things happen. When Sarah says *wah wah*, her version of *water*, she gets the real stuff. Her early experience with talking tells her that saying a word will make the real thing appear. (I can't help but believe that these early talking times give us the feeling that somehow if we say something it will happen, and makes us reluctant to express our fears lest they should become a reality. Of course Sarah does not yet have a realistic notion of how things do happen, of the relationship between cause and effect.)

Play Speech (Jargon)

You notice that sometimes Sarah chatters away and you can't make head or tail of what she is saying. You might even be worried because you know she can say a few words and yet she seems to forget the words she knows and lapse into gibberish. This is normal—it is play talk. Sarah has to practice not only her words but the other aspects of speech: fluency and tone of voice. She is not skilled enough in saying her words, nor does she have enough words to say to put them together for fluency, so she dispenses with real words (which are hard) and makes up nonsense speech to practice with. You may be amused to detect your own tone of voice in her play speech. Some parents are embarrassed to hear their own less than well mannered expression in their baby's play speech. Relax. You should accept it and enjoy it for what it is—"pretend" speech.

The Beginning of Grammar

When will Sarah put her words together and say sentences? To Sarah single words *are* sentences. Her speech may be a bit telegraphic, but by knowing the situation you understand the sentence she means to say. For example the word *out* to us would only be a fragment of a sentence and by itself would not communicate much. Sarah, however, uses the word *out* to mean a variety of related sentences having to do with the idea of outside the house. Because you know the situation you can understand the rest of the sentence when Sarah says "Out." "Look out the window," "I went out," "I want to go out," "I will go out," "You are going out," "I don't want to go out," "I left it outside." All of these sentences are possible meanings of the single word. Gesture and situation can make up for the lack of grammar. You can help Sarah to the next step in learning to talk by supplying the complete sentence for her when she uses a single word to express herself. You know what the complete sentence is, so you can say it. If there is noise in the street and Sarah says "Out" while pointing out the window, you can say "Look out the window." You don't expect her to repeat the adult form of the sentence, but at least she is hearing it. As Sarah is having her coat buttoned, she might say "Out." Then you can say: "Put your coat on to go out."[4]

Helping Your Child to Understand New Words

When you give Sarah a word she hasn't yet used, combine it with a gesture which will make it easier to understand. For instance, "It is cold" can be said holding your arms and making a shivering motion. Many parents naturally combine gestures with words: shaking the head sideways while saying "no," nodding the head up and down while saying "yes," waving while saying "bye bye," holding out the arms while saying "big" or "so big." Some people use gestures in everyday speech more than others. If you are a person not given to gesturing as you talk, try to do more of it to help your baby understand words.

Early Attempts at Pronunciation

Soon after her first word at about a year, you notice that Sarah's vocabulary is growing and almost every day you hear new words. These words are not pronounced perfectly. In spite of the months of mouth practice Sarah's first efforts are only approximations of a word. Since you have to have a sympathetic ear and bend your expectations of the English language a bit, you can hear *kacko* as *cracker* and *Tattytaw* as *Santa Claus*. Notice that the consonants M, P, B, T, D, N, H, Y and W are Sarah's most used sounds. The S and Z and CH and SH are harder to say, so Sarah replaces them with one of the sounds she can say.[5] Thus *salt* could become *talt*, *sister* becomes *titter* (easy T for harder S) or *zoo* is

4. Bloom and Lahey (1978). It may not be accurate to say that the single-word utterance is a sentence, but it translates into an adult sentence. The linguistically missing information is in the context and situation. Sometimes there will be two separate words which are not related grammatically, such as "car Billy," which is simply naming behavior and not to be confused with two-word sentences such as "mama gone."

5. H. Winitz, *From Syllable to Conversation* (Baltimore: University Park Press, 1975). Early attempts at pronouncing words are approximations of the adult production. If you trace the evolution of a word the production changes month by month but not always closer to the adult production. Perhaps the retention of these approximate but not mature pronunciations can be the beginning of articulation problems.

said *doo* (D for Z). *Chicken* is likely to be *ticken*, and *jam* would sound like *dam* or *yam*.

You are not Sarah's speech teacher. Do not teach her the specific words *you* think she should know. She will learn the words she needs as she becomes aware of her need for them during her second year. Your contribution is to be ready to supply the words. Encourage and support her efforts at speech. Learning to talk may be one of the most intellectually taxing accomplishments a person ever undertakes. Sarah needs to keep experimenting, keep trying without fear of failure. If you correct her pronunciation before she is ready to tackle difficult sounds, are unrealistic about her ability to succeed, and show your disapproval at her inevitable failure in achieving adult standards, you supply her with the main barrier to learning—fear of failure, which leads to a disinclination to try. Sarah has to keep trying to learn and the best way is for her not to be concerned with the possibility of failure. Never correct her by saying, "No, that's not the way to say it, say ____." If you catch a mispronunciation, insert the word into your regular conversation several times, prolonging the troublesome parts so that she can build up a sound image of the word.

Sometimes the effort of producing words becomes too cumbersome a means of communication and the child tries to substitute another method such as gesture. Although pairing the gesture with the word was a handy way to aid Sarah in understanding new words, do not let the gesture become the substitute for her attempt to say the word; that is, do not always respond to her gestures unless she has tried to accompany them with words. If a child points to a toy out of reach and that is enough to get the parent to get the toy down, there is no incentive to going to the trouble to say the difficult word. Don't be smart all the time; you don't always have to understand and respond to gestures.

Imitation

By the time Sarah is a year and a half old you realize that your child is full of surprises. It is tax paying time in your home. Sarah is playing on the floor by herself, presumably oblivious to your concern of the moment, filling out your tax return. As you discuss the various fine points of your return, you hear Sarah say "De-du'ion." You go on, thinking you are imagining things. Then a few minutes later, "Dedu'ion, dedu'ion." She really did say deduction! What kind of word is that for a baby? How could she know it? Is she some kind of genius? The taxes are forgotten for a moment as Sarah repeats her wonderful word. No, the word *deduction* is not really part of her vocabulary at all. Occasionally babies pick up words they hear and reproduce them without being aware of their meaning. She is practicing imitating the sound of your words. This echoing or parroting back (echolalia is the technical term) is part of the normal learning of speech. Sometimes it is amusing as the child produces a surprising word. At other times it is frustrating. You ask your child a question and instead of an answer you get the question back. "Where is your cap?" you ask. Sarah replies "Where is your cap?" This is not communication but speech practice for your child. Your problem is that you thought you were trying to communicate. You can expect this parroting of your speech before Sarah is two. It will go away as Sarah becomes better at talking and communicating.

Two and Three Years

Language Helps Your Baby to Learn

Language not only serves as communication but helps children understand their experiences—what they see and what is happening around them. Children learn what their role should be in the world through use of language. But understanding the behavior of persons and things and one's interactions with them obviously requires more than one word to complete a thought: there must be a reference to whatever you are talking about or are concerned with (usually a noun) or whatever it does and how it behaves or what you do to it (a verb). Dolly fall. Doggie run. Daddy come. These are examples of early attempts at putting words together to form sentences. When parents do the listening there is less guessing and less need to know the complete situation in order to understand what the child is saying. Sometimes a simple sentence will describe something: "Kitty soft" or "Dolly pretty." The child is not only aware of these things but observing their characteristics. The attribute "soft" will be applied to a kitten or a pillow or a teddy bear or a lap. You will notice that your child puts these words together in different combinations and thus displays the truly creative nature of human language. Even with a limited vocabulary it is possible to put words together to say something new, something that you have never heard anyone else say before. You can express a thought that is all your own. At about two years you notice this beginning attempt at grammar. Sarah is just two when this conversation occurs:

>MOTHER: See the little puppy?
>SARAH: Pitti [pretty] puppy.
>MOTHER: Be careful, don't hurt the puppy.
>SARAH: No hurt puppy.
>MOTHER: Careful! [Sarah's fingers are in the puppy's eye] Puppy
>will bite you.
>SARAH: Ow! No bite puppy.
>MOTHER: Pet him like this. [demonstrates]
>SARAH: [petting puppy] Ni' [nice] puppy. Look puppy kiss.
>MOTHER: That's because the puppy loves you.
>SARAH: No bite puppy lub [love] puppy. No hurt puppy.

The puppy and mother were teaching Sarah the proper treatment of puppies. Dogs use the disciplinary nip to teach their own kind how to behave; mothers use words to teach their children. The child will remember because of the words as much as the event of the little bite. Sometime later you hear your child talking to the new puppy: "No bite puppy, Sarah puppy lub." You realize that Sarah was internalizing this behavioral rule; that is, beginning to understand the consequence of her actions. A nip is the result of putting a finger in the puppy's eye and a lick or dog kiss is the result of petting. Moreover, she is remembering which result she wanted, therefore which action is preferable. This lesson and many more like it need to be repeated before the rule is internalized permanently. It is unreasonable for a parent to expect behavior from a child which cannot be explained simply enough to be understood by that child.

Learning "Good" Grammar

At three years Sarah's sentences become more and more complex and you are puzzled by some of the mistakes in grammar you hear. One month you hear "Birdie flew away" and "Daddy came home." These are grammatical constructions Sarah hears at home, and you are not at all surprised. The next month, however, Sarah says "Birdie flied away" and "Daddy comed home." She has certainly not heard sentences like *that* at home. What has happened?

She is learning grammar. She is not learning it the way we did in school, but learning it without realizing it—the way we all know grammar. We just know how to put the words together to say exactly what we mean. Sarah has picked up the rule for how you change an action into something that happened before (past tense). You add the *ed*, and for the most part this does the trick. It is a sign of progress that Sarah has internalized the rule of expressing the past tense and is applying it every time she needs to express something that happened before. This is not imitation but a logical application of the rule. She was tripped up by the exceptions in our language where the rule does not apply and a different sound is needed. You need not worry: Sarah will internalize the modifications of the rule the same way she internalized the rule in the first place. It just so happens that the words we use most often and therefore most likely to be learned by young children are the words most likely to have irregular endings. *Man, woman, child* have irregular plurals and *eat, drink, run, come, go, put* and *sleep* have irregular tense endings. So at this stage we may hear *mans, womans, childs, eated, drinked, runned, comed, goed, putted, sleeped* and other constructions of this type.

Scrambled Word Order

You may also notice that at two to three years Sarah puts her words in unusual order in her sentences: "Mommy no bed go Sarah," "Me no like carrots," "Billy me no want play." In the first two sentences you can be pretty sure of the meanings. Sarah is telling Mommy that she (Sarah) does not wish to go to bed. She is probably not telling her mother that she (mother) should not go to bed. In the second it is pretty clear how Sarah feels about carrots. What about the third sentence? Is she saying that she does not want to play with Billy? Or is she saying that Billy does not want to play with her? Here is an instance in which her primitive syntax failed to communicate precisely what she meant. Some frustration over misunderstanding of this kind must surely act as an impetus to modify grammar, making it conform more to the adult form. You can help Sarah at this stage to change her grammar to an understandable form. Without seeming to correct her you can simply repeat what she has said, changing it to standard grammar. When Sarah says, "Car no go" you can say, "The car won't go." Avoid saying to her "No, say the car won't go." That sounds punitive, and you don't want to punish Sarah for experimenting with language, a necessity for learning it. If you want to get across the idea of correction as a means of modifying speech, correct yourself in Sarah's presence: "Me no find keys. No, I can't find my keys. I just can't find my keys." You are using Sarah's type of baby grammar (although not a specific sentence she said) and correcting yourself. There is no penalty to Sarah, but there is some instruction. It gives Sarah an example of how one can listen to oneself and change what one has said to a more desirable form. Be sure to emphasize the correct form so as not to cause confusion over which is the correct model.

Playing with the Sound of Words

The preschool years can be wonderfully interesting for the parent who is aware of and involved with the child's learning process. Between two and three years you might notice that Sarah plays with rhyming words much the way she played with syllables in her first year. If she thinks no one is around you may hear nonsense poems like "pappy, sappy, happy, fappy." This may sound silly to you, but it is merely Sarah in her word laboratory experimenting with the sound of words. The meanings are explored as they change with little sound changes. Rhyming may also act as a memory aid for Sarah. Cultures without a written language (Sarah has no writing yet) commit their history to memory and in order to aid that memory put it into poetry, which is easier to remember than prose. Nursery rhymes will be appreciated now. Sarah won't know the meaning, but she will like the sound. Most of us don't know the meaning of nursery rhymes (who knows what a tuffet is except that Miss Muffet sat on it?). They have lasted so long that I feel they have been used by children over the centuries, not to tell a story but to practice the free flow of speech. They are strings of words that are easy to remember and say over and over.

Where Things Are

At around three years Sarah discovers that all the parts of the body have names and she is busy learning them. With the name goes the conscious awareness of the body part itself. Of course babies "discover" the parts of their bodies long before this. But with words this discovery becomes knowledge on a new level. For instance, the shoulder was there all along but Sarah couldn't have said how her arms were connected with her body until that part was named. At this age Sarah begins to relate objects to each other in space. She needs prepositions to do this. The sock can be *on* the bed or it can be *under* the bed or it can be *in* the drawer. These little words make a lot of difference when you want to find the sock. Play games with her. At first say "Put the ball *in* the box" while you put the ball in the box. Then give the ball to Sarah and say "You put the ball *in* the box." This could be the beginning of help in household tasks. "Put the towel *in* the hamper." Accompanying the words with the actions makes it easier for Sarah to learn the words.

Combining Words with Pictures

Reading stories while looking at the pictures of the story is another way to combine words with actions. For Sarah at three a really good book is a story that stands alone without the words (the pictures are complete) and in which the printed words stand alone without the pictures. Thus Sarah can experience the story by listening to the words as you read them and by looking at the pictures by herself. You may find Sarah "reading" a favorite book by herself, looking at the pictures and saying the story out loud, combining words with action.

When Sarah has passed her third birthday her speech should be understood by strangers. You probably still find some mispronounced words, but they won't be so frequent nor so peculiar that people can't understand her at all. She uses many more words than she used a few months earlier. Remember, too, that she knows and understands many more words than she says. This is true for all of us. We all know more spoken words than we actually use, and we all have larger reading vocabularies than writing vocabularies. There will be an interval between the time Sarah learns a word and the time she ventures to say it.

Personal Pronouns

At this time Sarah is learning to use *I* when referring to herself rather than *me* or *Sarah*. The proper use of the personal pronouns may not seem a big accomplishment to you but it can be mind-boggling to a three-year-old.

FATHER: I roll the ball to you, Sarah.

SARAH [as the ball is rolling toward her]: Ball roll to you.

FATHER: No, not to me, to you.

SARAH: Yes, to you.

FATHER: When *I* say you, I mean *you*, Sarah. When I say I, I mean *me*, Daddy.

SARAH: I, Sarah.

FATHER: OK, you roll the ball to me.

SARAH [rolling ball to father]: You roll the ball to me.

FATHER: *No*, you are rolling the ball to me.

SARAH: Yeah, you roll to me.

This will get straightened out with time. When Sarah wants to make sure that the person she is talking to knows that she is talking about herself she will use the word *me*, or to really make sure, use her name, Sarah. From hearing her parents and others using pronouns, she will figure out that she should say *I* when she is talking about herself and others use *I* only when talking about themselves. It is a pesky set of words which can change meaning depending upon who is saying them.

Nonliteral Language

Another way to help your child acquire grammar is to use correct but simple grammatical forms. Long complicated sentences tax your child's comprehension and memory span. One thought at a time is enough. "See the big fierce-looking brown dog running down the street toward the Jones's house" is just too much for the two- to three-year-old child to take in all at once. You have said that there is a dog, that it is big, that it is brown, that it is fierce- (whatever that means) looking (who is looking, the dog or you? Or does looking mean something else in this sentence?). It is running down (down is toward your feet) the street and is also going in the direction of the Jones's house. (Bobby's house?) You avoid talking like this to your child because you instinctively know that there is too much information all at once and that such a sentence provides a confusing—even incomprehensible—model for your child to learn from.

There are many confusions you take for granted in our language that are not obvious to the two- or three-year-old. Sarah may know that she has a head and that you have a head, but it is hard for her to see the head of a table. How can a stove or a needle

have eyes? If you say "Don't be a wet blanket" that is ridiculous—
no person can be a wet blanket to the literal-minded two- and
three-year-old. Sarah has to learn not only the literal meanings of
words but their colloquial and idiomatic meanings. When we say
the road winds along the valley and the river runs along beside it,
we are using an expanded meaning of the words *wind* and *run*.
When we hear the language that we have taken for granted for so
long with the unsophisticated comprehension of a small child we
can realize its richness and complexity.[6] There is no point for a
parent to try to expunge all idioms from the language. If you
recognize the problem and add some extra explanation the learning task will be made easier. Sarah will have to learn all these
things as you have, but at her own pace as you did.

Broad and Narrow Meanings of Words

Another problem the three-year-old has with the language is
that the words the child uses do not have the precision of meaning
that the same words have when used by an adult. Sarah at three
calls all animals dogs. Elephants, mice, cows—in fact anything on
four legs—is a dog. Can't she see the difference between a dog and
a cow and a mouse? She probably can but does not think the
distinction is important enough to take into account. She really
means to say four-legged animal when talking about these creatures. To Sarah, a dog is a general class of creature, but no one ever
gave her the suitable words for the class, quadruped, so she makes
do with the first word she did learn for a four-legged animal, dog.
You misunderstand her because when you hear the word, *dog*, you
think it is the particular animal. Sarah signaled that she was ready
to differentiate the various four-legged animals when she started
needing modifiers for dog. At the zoo the lion was named *big dog*
and the elephant was named *big big dog*. Realizing that the time
for naming has come and understanding why all the animals had
been dogs before, you explain that although the lion looks something like a big dog it is called a lion. Later Sarah will learn that all
reading matter is not to be called a book. A book is one type of

6. Normal children like Sarah learn to deal with nonliteral meanings surprisingly
early, perhaps indicating that most human beings have an inborn ability in metaphor.
But a language-delayed child or language-disordered child may continue to have difficulty with terms such as "running water" or "green with envy."

reading matter; magazines and newspapers are other kinds. When we give a child a word for a particular thing such as a clock, the child may take that word to mean that class of things and call every kind of timepiece from the timer on the stove to a wristwatch a clock. As the child gets older the meanings of the words become more particularized.

Four to Six Years

Thinking Out Loud

Children often talk to themselves because they have not yet learned to use words without actually saying them as we do when we think to ourselves. If you listen without being patronizing and judgmental you can eavesdrop on your child's thinking. You may get a ringside seat to Sarah's attempts to organize her world. You may be amused to hear Sarah ordering herself around and obeying her orders. "Put the pail away." Then she puts the toy pail in the toy box. Is she reflecting being ordered around by adults? Or is she just putting her intentions into words and, instead of thinking them to herself, saying them out loud? Probably a bit of both. This is another example of a child putting together words and actions. "Dolly a bad girl. Make a mess. Spill milk all over. Mama mad." She is not only reliving some incident by remembering it and learning from it, but is also accepting what may have been a painful experience.

Parents whose children have had surgery or who have been badly frightened in an accident report that their children often act out the event over and over in their play. Language is a means of communication and the medium of thinking, but it has a third function of expressing and coming to grips with emotion. The reliving of the fearful can even fade away the horror through familiarity. Since the event probably frightened the parents too, they hope it will be quickly forgotten and life can resume as if it had never happened. They are distressed to find their child stubbornly reenacting it and refusing to forget it. By reliving the event the child turns the unknown experience (which is why it was so frightening in most cases) into a known and therefore less frightening one. People (including young children) have language as a means with which to think about and come to terms with these events.

Language and Anticipation

Just as language can help your child remember and relive the past, it can also anticipate the future. For the very young, such as Sarah at two or three, the future is no more than a few hours off. Probably the idea of Christmas won't have much meaning for Sarah in October. She will either think it is tomorrow or will conceive of a future event in the same way that we do when we think of the sun cooling down—as something incredibly far away in time. Grandma's visit tomorrow is quite a lot of anticipation. The use of the future is one of the last grammatical constructions learned by children. When the idea of the future is understood, Sarah learns and understands the use of the future tense and eventually includes it in her language.

Help Sarah understand anticipation by keeping the time between the anticipated event and the present short when she is two and three years old. "We will go to the park after your nap." The nap is over, and sure enough you go out to the park. Be careful to see that the anticipated event actually happens. As Sarah gets older the time of anticipation can be stretched. Often parents overestimate how long a child can look forward to something. Even at six years of age, a child probably can only anticipate an event two weeks away. A structured life in which events happen in a fairly orderly and predictable manner is probably a help for a child learning the concept of the future. Some children demand an elaborate bedtime ritual which is the same every night. This seems to give them the security of knowing that what they expect to happen actually does happen. Even if Sarah's life is very structured, however, the future is not so sure as the past. You might say it is going to rain this afternoon and then the rain fails to materialize. With hindsight you can admit your prediction was wrong: "I thought when I got up that it was going to rain." Sarah also needs to learn that things don't always happen as anticipated.

Imaginary and Real Events

With language you can describe an event that never happened and perhaps could not happen. This is the basis of fantasy. The anticipated event may be the first experiment with thinking about something that did not happen, as it hasn't happened yet. But you and Sarah will move on to stories and dreams and wishes. "Let's pretend we had a chocolate cake as big as a bus—what would we do?" "Suppose that cats could talk." The stories you read and tell to Sarah will expand and exercise her imagination. She can try on different realities just as she sees herself in different clothes when she plays "dress-up." At four Sarah starts to understand that there is a difference between those "let's pretend" and "suppose that" events and the everyday events of her life. When she uses the *would be* rather than the *is* to describe these events she is on her way to understanding the difference. Some children have difficulty sorting out the real from the imaginary. By school age the imaginary should be reliably separated from the real.

Before Sarah has made the distinction between the real and the imaginary she can have real fears of imaginary monsters. Her verbal skills create a monster that lurks under her bed and even though she realizes that she has made it up she is not at all sure that it couldn't exist. You may think you reassure her by telling her that a monster she made up couldn't possibly be real. But she may not realize how limited her creative powers are. If she can have its image in her mind, the way she can have images of family members in her mind, it might be real. Moreover, her monster may be psychologically useful to her in teaching her how to cope with fear. We all carry some of this apprehension of our own imagination with us throughout our lives. We do not want to name a feared or terrible thing. If we put words to it and say them out loud, we make it more real and somehow more probable.

The confusions and apprehensions brought on by anticipation of the future, separating real and imaginary events and fearing the products of our own imagination are a part of learning language. No one can say for sure whether our language deals with these things because this is the way our minds work, or if our minds have these confusions because our language develops them. At any rate while Sarah is growing up you will be aware of some of the things her mind is cooking up and you can help her by your understanding and reassurance.

The Greatest Learning Time of Life

The preschool years are the greatest learning years in a person's life. Never again will a person experience such a knowledge explosion. How can you be sure your child makes the most of these productive learning years? Your child will talk more if there is plenty to talk about. Your child will learn more if exposed to a rich and stimulating life. Your child is learning by direct experience: seeing a variety of colors, smelling different smells, tasting different tastes, doing a wide range of things. What looks like play to you is really your child's job. It is a serious career. Provide your child with puzzles, games, toys, other children and other adults. The toys need not be expensive nor declared educational by some expert. A bucket of sand and a shovel and some containers can provide a learning experience. Add some water to this and there is a whole new learning experience. Modelling clay can be bought or made from water, salt and soda. Your child can learn that the same wad of clay can be formed into a pancake and then reformed into a snake. Dolls aid your child in acting out stories or events that happened at home. Your child needs to see other people besides your immediate family. The experience of making oneself understood by the not so forgiving ear of a stranger helps in getting your child to improve pronunciation and become familiar with the speech of others. Reading books to your child reveals their pleasures and, since the school years coming up will be full of books, developing a love of books will be an advantage. Read books and stories to your child, preferably books with pictures so that your child is "reading" with you.

Do not try to teach your child to read before school. Your child may not be ready for it; the difference between the letters is not always easy for a child to see. There is no point in trying something at a time when chances for success are small. Moreover, I do not suggest the early teaching of reading because reading is a derived experience. Even if your child can master the skill of reading, it is better to have smelled a rose before reading about it. It is also better to perfect the spoken language, which the written language is based upon, as the foundation for reading.

Take your child places. Shopping is fascinating and stimulating. Instead of feeling that you are dragging the child along because you have to do errands and there is no one to stay home, look on these times as an opportunity to expand your child's world. Give your child some chore such as carrying a small sack in order to feel useful and needed. Talk to your child about what you are doing and why you are doing it. For instance, "Here is the hamburger—we can have some hamburger for dinner." You might even remind your child later at dinner that this is the hamburger you bought together.

Talk with your child about the day's events. If your child has been at day care or at nursery school listen to what has happened. Often parents don't really listen to their children's account of events. If you listen and ask questions when something is not clear, you help your child learn to tell a coherent account of an event.

Even though your child's life is full of varied and stimulating experiences, try to keep the excitement from getting out of hand. Routine is very reassuring for a small child. Some disruptions of routine are inevitable, but a largely unpredictable life makes a child feel uncertain. The child may come to feel that life cannot be organized or controlled at all. The child with a more structured life is better able to branch out and look at new things. Language is a way of structuring the events that happen and the structured life reflects the structure of language.

Now is the time to teach Sarah her last name. By four years most children know their full names. One of my earliest memories is being taught my last name and how to spell it before I even knew what the letters were. Soon afterward you should teach Sarah your address as a safety measure.

As Sarah's vocabulary increases, she begins to sort the words she knows into categories. You can help her organize her words through word games. She is still too young to understand a competitive game, one where there is a winner and a loser, but will love cooperative games. Start by saying, "How many things to eat can you think of? I'll start with apples and eggs." Together you can build up a list of foods. You may want to refine it later to fruits or to breakfast foods or foods you like and so forth. Another game can be to think of all you can wear and name them. This game can be refined to what you wear in the summertime or what you wear on Sunday, etc. These games are great for car trips.

The year from four to five is also a good year for puppets. Children use puppets both to express themselves and to listen to. I have seen children who could not understand directions for a task given by an adult understand the same directions given by a puppet. You don't have to be a skilled ventriloquist to be a successful puppeteer with your child. The puppet can say "Pick up your toys and get ready for bed" and get better results than you can without the puppet on your hand. Some shy children feel threatened by the concentrated one-on-one contact with an adult and seem to feel easier talking through a puppet. Some of your word games may be more successful using a puppet.

After the fourth birthday your child is very much a person and a personality. She will use longer words and more of them. Sarah's words will be more precise. "I stubbed my toe" instead of "I hurt my foot." Both the event and the part of the body are more clearly expressed. Not only are her descriptions of things and happenings more precise, but she uses purely abstract words such as *glad* and *fun* and *mad* and *scary*. These feelings cannot be described at all with concrete objects. Her world has expanded and she needs to use her talking in many different situations. You find that her sense of time is greatly enlarged. When you go on an outing, plan with her what you are going to do. She will enjoy the planning and discover that looking forward is part of the fun of the treat if the time span is short enough. Talk to her about what you and she did. She can tell someone who was not on the outing about it. Encourage her to tell about things that happened. It is very good practice for her. A four-year-old's account of a trip to a department store may not be the most fascinating tale to listen to. But your child's accomplishment of putting together a coherent narrative *is* fascinating.

At this age television will have more meaning for Sarah, and you will be tempted to let her watch while you do other things. Some television shows are valuable and amusing for her, but mostly television does not aid speech development. The TV has too much noise, too much color, and too much happens faster than it can be taken in by a child. You will have noticed that Sarah's speaking and comprehension rate is slower than that of adults. Television is a one-way experience that doesn't care whether you understand or even listen to it. Children need to develop a two-way relationship to learn the social activity of talking. The television talks *at* children, not *to* them, and doesn't listen at all. It would be much better for Sarah if she could do the things herself instead of watching other children do things on some children's TV program. Reading books to Sarah may also seem like a derived experience, as is reading books to oneself. But when you read a book to a child, you are the magic ingredient. You are sharing and experiencing the story together. You are both in control of it. You can stop and talk about what is happening. The child can respond to what is happening and the person reading the story aloud listens to that response.

The games available to Sarah as she approaches her fifth birthday are more varied and complex. Try sound-of-word games as well as category-of-word games. For instance how many words start with *b* (pronounced *buh* not *bee*)? You can add to the list: baby, bear, big, blue, bubble etc. Sarah doesn't need the letters of the alphabet yet but learning to hear the sounds at the start of words is a good foundation for learning the alphabet, not only the letters but what they stand for in words and how they can be rearranged to form new words. I still would not push the written word at this point; Sarah may not be ready to learn her letters until she is six. But she is ready for sound and word play.

Sarah is now able to participate in various family projects and chores. You probably think that fall clean-up and raking leaves is dull, but Sarah doesn't know that, and her attempts to help may be fun for her and present the chore in a new light for you. There is always something she will be able to do. Children who are active participants in their family's doings seem to be more advanced in language. It may be that encouraging generally mature behavior spills over into more mature language. It could also be that participating in family tasks provides a greater opportunity for conversation with adults.

When you finally send Sarah off to first grade, you may think that this is the beginning of her education. But it is only the beginning of her formal education. She has learned much at home. She has mastered the difficult skill of producing all the speech sounds in all the combinations to form words. She has learned and continues to learn new words which stand for things, ideas, persons, attributes, conditions, actions, relationships. She has learned to put these words together to say precisely what she means. Although she will continue to elaborate and refine her grammar until she is about twelve, she has already developed most of it. Remember how she sounded when she started and listen to her now. At the beginning of her life, Sarah had no language at all. She was no more verbal than any wild animal, and certainly less competent to cope with the world than almost any animal. She developed her language, learned who she was, has a head full of culture, tradition and memories, all of which she accumulated from the particular language *you* gave her. Yes, it's true that she was designed to learn to talk from somebody. But she *did* learn to talk from *you*. Your contribution is a vital part of what makes her unique.

As Your Child Learns to Speak: Suggestions for Parents

- Hold and cuddle your infant while talking.
- Let your baby have time for vocal experimentation.
- Don't let your infant spend a large proportion of time awake crying. Noncrying awake time is speech and communication learning time.
- Talk to your child about what is happening even before the child could possibly understand.
- Remember the tone of voice is more important than the words to your baby.
- Use gestures with words to facilitate understanding.
- Describe in words what your child is doing in play.
- Describe in words what you are doing as your baby watches.
- Keep your sentences short, simple and correct.
- Don't expect perfect pronunciation in the beginning.
- Don't be too understanding of nonverbal communication. Wait until you notice an attempt to say the word before you understand.
- Don't correct poor grammar or pronunciation, just be sure you supply the correct model for your child to hear.
- Give your child a variety of toys and playthings.
- Take your child to a variety of places.
- Read books and/or tell stories to your child.
- Talk with your child about the day's events at the end of the day and talk about the day's plans at the beginning of the day.
- Listen to your child.

2

If Your Baby Doesn't Learn to Talk:
An Overview of Communication
Problems of Children

- *Speech Output Problems Without Physical Cause*
- *Speech Output Problems from Known Physical Causes*
- *Language Formation Problems*
- *Combination of Problems*
- *Recognizing Speech Language and Hearing Problems*

Sarah is six years old. You have just taken her to school for the first time, the beginning of her formal education. You remember when you first took her home from the hospital, a tiny helpless baby whose only sound was crying and whose only activity was eating. Now she is a poised articulate child who can carry on an intelligent conversation and can communicate her wishes, her likes and dislikes to you in clearly understood words. She is very much a person. You are a bit awed at the progress your little girl has made. And yet it is the normal course of development for the human child. Do all children develop this way? Most do, but not all. Considering the vastness of the accomplishment of going from baby to competent six-year-old, one is surprised that so many children do develop without problems.

School activities and the classroom curriculum are based upon past experience of what Sarah and other children her age have accomplished and learned before entering kindergarten. Sarah has learned all the different sounds of her language; she can form and understand about forty-four of them. At school she will learn to put the sounds she hears and forms together with the symbols she reads and writes, the twenty-six letters of the alphabet. The letters

would be meaningless if she had not learned the sounds they represent.[1] Sarah has also learned to assemble these forty-four sounds
into a few thousand words. Each word stands for an object, an
action, a quality, an abstract characteristic, a relationship and so
forth. These words are the vocabulary of her education. But individual words are not enough. She has learned to assemble them to
express fine nuances of meaning. The words enable her to talk
about and understand things that happened in the past, are happening right now, that will happen in the future, and things that
never did and never will happen except in the imagination. She
has learned the rules of grammar, not consciously in order to describe them, but unconsciously in order to use them. All academic
learning is based upon these skills.

Language is also the basic tool for social relationships and development. Sarah will make new friends, and these friendships will
start with talking. Through speech she learns what is acceptable
behavior in school and on the playground. She demonstrates who
she is, her character, intelligence and personality, in her group of
friends by what she says. Thus anything that goes wrong with this
communication process could have a devastating effect on a child's
whole life. Even supposedly minor problems encountered by children learning to talk can be very distressing to parents and the
child.

Speech Output Problems Without Physical Cause

Unclear Speech (Articulation Problems)

Some children have trouble forming the sounds they hear.
When five-year-old Becky speaks, her speech is obviously different. She says, for example, "Witto Wed Widing Hood" instead of
"Little Red Riding Hood." A careful listener can understand her
but Becky sounds "funny." She has not learned to produce all the
sounds she needs for clear speech. This is the most common speech
problem in young children. There are varying estimates ranging

1. There are approximately forty-four different meaningful speech sounds (pho-
nemes) in American English, twenty-five consonants and fifteen vowels and four diph-
throngs. Different dialects may have different numbers of sounds. For instance, many
people never say the *wh* sound, pronouncing "where" and "wear" the same way. Certain
regions have their own vowel variations, and there are sounds in dialects outside the U.S.
not ever found in General American.

from six million children with this type of disorder to 2 to 3 percent or 120,000 to 180,000 of all elementary schoolchildren who
have severe pronunciation problems. A severe form of this problem is speech so unclear that a sympathetic listener or even family
member cannot understand it. There are probably many more
children with milder speech sound problems who still can be understood. This problem of mispronunciation may clear up by itself,
but some mispronunciations persist. The longer a child mispronounces words the stronger the habit of mispronunciation becomes
and the harder it is to correct. Becky might be able to hear the
difference between the R and the W in others' speech and therefore would be able to learn the letter R and the letter W. Her
difficulty arises when her attempt to produce a good R in *red* fails
and results in W as in *wed*. She knows the difference but cannot
produce it because she has not learned to move her tongue properly.[2]

Some children fail to hear the differences in speech sounds.
This problem can cause extreme difficulty in learning to read because the letters do not make sense to a child who has not learned
to listen to the sounds. Marcus's speech is very hard to understand.
He leaves off the ends of words completely and mispronounces
many of the beginnings. When he says "Sing a Song of Sixpence"
it sounds like "Tih uh taw uh tih puh." Marcus also says "Wun two
buto my too" for "One two buckle my shoe." When you look at
Marcus's speech pattern you see that he uses the T sound where he
should use the S (in *sing*), but he also uses the T for the CK sound
(in *buckle*) and the SH (in *shoe*) as well as in the right place (in
two). For a child like Marcus, what does the letter T on a page
mean? He needs to pair the sounds he hears with the letters he
sees. But if the sounds he is using are confused how can he sort out
the letters? Marcus may hear better than he speaks, but there is no
way for his parents or teachers to be sure. Furthermore a child
who confuses the S in *sing* with the T in *two* with the SH in *shoe*
and the CK in *buckle* may not be ready to see the differences in
the letters S, CK, T and SH. On the other hand Marcus could be
one of those visually oriented children who have an easier time
sorting out the sounds when the visual representation is in front of

2. There are some authorities in the field who say the RSL problems will mostly
clear up on their own and are due to immature speech mechanism. Such a problem is
easier to dismiss if it is not happening to your own child.

them. Whatever the nature of his problem, Marcus is entering school at a disadvantage.

Unclear speech is a social as well as communication disadvantage. Even if spared an academic penalty, however, there is a social penalty which is very costly to such children. A ten-year-old boy, for instance, with a lisp (thalty thoup for salty soup) suffers taunts from his classmates for talking "funny." The psychological and social damage from one little mispronounced sound can seem disproportionate but should be taken into consideration by the parents. In general there is less tolerance for an older child than for a younger one who has this type of problem. When you hear an adult with this type of speech difficulty you tend to be more negative in your judgment of that person than you would for a child with the problem. You seldom find an adult with a pronunciation problem in the professions or in occupations which require talking to the public. People with unclear speech are more likely to be found in unskilled or semiskilled jobs. They are vocationally as well as socially handicapped by their speech. These adults may be intelligent and talented people, but no one has bothered to listen to what they have to say because of how they say it. Chapter 5 describes this kind of disorder in detail and how you as parents can help your child overcome it and also how the problem can be prevented in some cases.

Stuttered Speech

Another type of speech problem is getting the words to come out in a smooth flow of speech. The words by themselves may be pronounced correctly, but the rhythm is halting or jerky and sometimes the speech seems completely blocked. The child, fearful of these breaks in speech, struggles to avoid them. This combination of breaks in the rhythm of speech and the struggle to avoid them creates what we know as stuttering. Stumbling over speech is not always a permanent handicap, however. Robert at five stumbles over his words especially when he is excited. "L l l l l l look [deep breath]—Mmmmmmmmmmmmommy a-a-a-a-a sssssssssssssnake!" He may learn to take these breaks in stride and, when his speech becomes more proficient, the breaks will diminish in intensity and frequency. Or he may become like Marilyn at sixteen who cannot talk to strangers and therefore will not make new friends. She dreads shopping, not because she doesn't like to get new things but because she is afraid she will freeze up and not be able to say anything when the salesperson asks, "Can I help you?" When she does talk she cannot look at the person she is talking to and seems to fight her own mouth to get the words out.

Stuttering, which occurs in about one in a hundred children, is a miserable handicap for those afflicted. To the nonstutterer, the rhythmic flow of speech does not seem the tremendous accomplishment it seems to the stutterer. But to the person who stutters, fluency can become a major goal in life. Stutterers will avoid certain speech situations, situations which they otherwise wish to be part of, in order to avoid the danger of the dreaded speech blocks. They will also avoid certain people, sometimes going to elaborate pains not to have to speak to them, since these people may react to the stutterer's struggle to get word out with impatience, embarrassment, condescension, contempt and even laughter. Few people would want to elicit these kinds of reactions when they speak to others. Chapter 8 describes stuttering, how parents can help to prevent it and, if it is already developed, how you can help your child control it.

Voice Problems: Medical, Psychological, Habitual

Children (as well as adults) often have a problem with the voice itself.[3] A child's voice may be too soft for you to hear. It could be caused by a medical dysfunction of the voice box (larynx) which in most cases can be cured with proper medical treatment. Sometimes the too soft voice happens with a healthy larynx. In such a case there may be a psychological reason. The child could be using the inaudible voice as a means of withdrawing from other people.

Voices are peculiar. A voice that is fine for one age and sex may sound totally inappropriate for another age and/or sex. Tony at twelve years old has clear fluent speech, but his voice is so high pitched he sounds like a very small child. This is particularly distressing to Tony because he is at an age in which he wants to present a more mature and masculine image. He may grow out of it in time, but his concerned parents want to find out what caused

3. There is not a special chapter on voice disorders in this book. Children do have voice problems, but they are often part of other communication or medical problems.

it and how they can help. He could have a naturally small and tight larynx which will change as he matures. He could also have a medical disorder. Before speech therapy is considered or begun, examination by a physician specializing in throat disorders is a must. Tony may be habitually tense. Everyone's voice rises when feeling nervous or tense. Tony could have adopted a falsetto voice without being aware of it to avoid the pitch breaks that often come with the beginning of adolescent voice change. Tony's parents can help him find his natural voice pitch by encouraging him to try to match his speaking voice to his nonspeaking vocalizations such as clearing his throat or grunting from muscular effort. Voice problems are not rare, but they are usually not brought to the attention of speech clinicians. Many people believe there is nothing to be done to improve the voice if it is too loud or too soft, too high pitched or too low pitched or is nasal, harsh, strident, breathy or husky. Any time a person's voice is so conspicuous that the listener is more concerned with the sound of the voice than what the speaker is saying, communication is impeded. Voice problems can be symptoms of disease or neurological problems and should not be ignored.

Speech Output Problems from Known Physical Causes

Cerebral Palsy

The stuttering and pronunciation problems described so far are habits of speech without a physical cause. Voice problems may or may not have a physical cause. Some children may have physical problems that affect their pronunciation or rhythm or voice quality or all three. Luis finally learned to talk. He has cerebral palsy and has difficulty controlling his movements, including his speech movements. He has trouble forming the more difficult sounds in words and so leaves out or replaces some of these hard sounds with other sounds he finds easier to say. For instance he calls himself 'uid instead of Luis. Sometimes he has a hard time organizing his speech movements. Pauses are followed by explosive blurting of speech that sounds somewhat like stuttering blocks in his talk. Sometimes he has difficulty controlling the pitch of his voice, and so his voice goes up and down the scale. Luis will be able to learn some control of his speech organs but his speech will always sound somewhat different. How to help your cerebral palsied child is discussed in Chapter 7.

Cleft Palate or Cleft Lip

Another speech output problem can arise when children are born with facial deformities. The most common of these is cleft lip and/or palate. Dora was born with a cleft palate and lip. Now that she is three the cleft has been repaired surgically, but she still has trouble closing off the back of her nose from her mouth. Normally when a person is not talking or eating, the nose and the mouth are connected. This is why it is possible to breathe through your nose with your mouth shut; the air goes through your nose down your throat and into the lungs. During eating, the air route from mouth to lungs must be closed so that you won't choke. Also the route from the nose to the mouth must be closed while you eat and most of the time when you talk. Your soft palate acts like a valve closing off the back of the nose from the mouth. You can see for yourself by opening your mouth in front of a well-lighted mirror and saying *aaah*. You should see the back of your palate jump up and back when you start saying *aaah*. For all the speech sounds except M, N and NG the soft palate must move this way. Normally when you speak your soft palate moves to close and open the nose rapidly. After all the surgery, Dora's soft palate still does not move so easily and rapidly as it should. If she is tired, which makes her soft palate even more sluggish, her voice takes on a nasal resonance which many people find unpleasant. Moreover Dora's tongue is not as mobile as it normally should be and her speech has a somewhat thick sound to it. Knowing about Dora's problem from the beginning, her parents make sure she receives the speech therapy she needs to speak more clearly and to improve her voice quality. They help her at home as well as take her to the clinic. They are aware that Dora is more likely to have ear infections and have learned that hearing loss from infections, even though temporary, can affect her speech development. Like Luis, Dora has many types of speech problems from one basic cause. How to help your child who has cleft palate or lip is discussed in Chapter 6.

Language Formation Problems

Becky, Marilyn, Luis and Dora are children who have trouble talking, but not in figuring out what they want to say. Their internal organization is normal, but the outward or vocal expression of their thoughts is impeded. For other children the language structure itself can be impaired. They are frustrated not because they are unable to express what they are thinking, but because they cannot verbalize their thoughts. In a sense they do not know what they are thinking before putting it into words. This distinction seems clear enough in theory but it is a hard one to make in any given case. As a parent or teacher, all you can understand of a child's language processes is what the child actually says. You may not be able to tell immediately if your child's disordered speech is the result of some impediment in the speech output or the result of impaired ability to form the language. Yet this distinction must be made in order to help your child. You need to know whether to help your child build a language or to facilitate the expression of the already built language. It doesn't make much sense to teach a child how to pronounce words correctly when the child neither knows their meanings nor is able to use them in communication.

Delayed Speech for No Apparent Reason

Woody left out most of the consonant sounds when he spoke. He said *'ah* for *car, 'ow* for *house* and *'a'* for *bath*. At four and a half his speech was unintelligible. The speech teacher in the day care center assumed Woody had a bad pronunciation problem. He had passed hearing screening so hearing loss was ruled out. Woody was put on a program of intensive articulation therapy in which he was trained to say the K, M, P and T sounds: first alone, then in nonsense syllables, then in words and finally in sentences. He was doing fine at the word level but failed at the sentence level. Nobody had noticed that Woody never talked in sentences at all. He had never used more than one word at a time to communicate. His problem was deeper than being unable to form certain consonant sounds. He knew only a few words and no sentence structure. The articulation therapy did not even touch his basic problem. He needed training in pairing words with objects and actions and then pairing events with simple sentences such as "Drop the ball" as the ball is dropped. Although it is not always possible to pinpoint the ultimate cause of a communication disorder, it is necessary to identify the nature of that disorder.

Some children have their senses intact and still do not develop a language, or do not develop a language at the rate other children do. Sometimes the problem seems to be that the child's mind does not process information delivered by the senses. A child may hear other people speaking; that is, be aware of the sound, but cannot understand it. This child lacks the ability to sort out the sounds of talking to decipher the message. Words once said are over very quickly and the child may not be able to figure out their meanings fast enough. When the words are combined with other words and come out rapidly one right after another, such a child has no way of managing this data overload and fails to understand what is being said. Although this may describe the nature of Woody's problem, no one can tell why Woody is not able to sort out speech sounds he hears. There is more detailed information on this problem in Chapter 3.

Delayed Speech from Hearing Loss or Deafness

If a child is not learning to speak at the expected age, the first thing to do is to see how well the child hears. Jeremy did not start to speak because he was unable to hear others speaking. Although his capacity for language was inborn and probably unimpaired, without being exposed to the speech of others he had no material with which to build his language. He needed to learn to understand as well as to learn to speak. If his hearing could have been miraculously restored overnight, he still would not have been able to communicate until he learned to understand and to speak, which would take some time. For more about the effect of hearing on speech see Chapter 4.

Delayed Speech from Learning Disabilities

Sometimes language delay goes with overall mental developmental delay (mental retardation). Learning is slower for these children, and so is learning to speak and understand. Moreover, these children do not spontaneously pick up language in many cases, but have to be taught it. Sometimes there is not an overall delay but a problem in one aspect of learning. This one difficulty can sometimes act as a "hang-up" for the whole language learning process. For example, if a child has a difficulty in sequencing or arranging things in the proper order, many aspects of language would be affected. The sounds in words must be in the prescribed order. The words in a sentence must be in a certain order for a specific meaning. There is a proper order to the information in telling a story, in giving directions, in all speech that communicates.

Mona spoke very strangely for a five-year-old child. Furthermore she did not seem to understand fully. She often seemed to understand part of the message, but she would mix things up. If her mother said, "Close the door," Mona might move toward the door or point to the door or simply repeat, "Close the door." She understood *door* but not what she was supposed to do with it. She spoke in sentences, but the sentences were often scrambled. "No Mommy want bed go" meant "I don't want to go to bed, Mommy." Mona had difficulty in sequencing. She knew the meanings of some words but she could not perceive them in the proper order nor could she seem to arrange them in the proper order to make her message clear. For instance, if Mona heard the sentence "Mickey is kissing Aunt Jill" she would not know whether Mickey was doing the kissing or Aunt Jill was doing the kissing. She can be helped to overcome this learning disability. Her parents and teachers must understand the precise nature of her problem (but not necessarily the cause) in order to help her overcome it. Mona can be shown the difference between "Mickey is kissing Aunt Jill" and "Aunt Jill is kissing Mickey." Chapter 3 discusses ways to help your learning-disabled child.

There are other specific difficulties labeled learning disabilities. Some of them, like Mona's, can affect speech and understanding; some can affect reading and writing. If the specific disability is understood, however, the child can receive special training in the weak area. Sometimes the problem can be circumvented. If a child, for instance, has a problem processing information taken in through hearing, the auditory information can be replaced and/or accompanied by the information coming in through a different sense such as pictures or gestures. It is unlikely that a normally hearing but learning disabled child would only use sign or gesture language for communication, but the child could use gesture as a bridge to learning auditory understanding of normal speech.

Delayed Speech from Known or Suspected Brain Damage

When a child is delayed in learning to talk there is often a suspicion of brain damage. The damage to the brain is not always easy to identify. A car accident in which a child suffered a severe head wound, after which the child's language seemed disordered, would point to an acquired language problem. But sometimes there is no history of accident or injury and yet the child acts as if there had been such an injury. The child may have behavioral symptoms of brain damage without anyone knowing when or if such damage occurred. It is often so slight that there are no clinical neurological tests sensitive enough to find it. Therefore the damage or dysfunction is only inferred from observing the child's behavior. There are many signs and symptoms with this situation: distractability, impulsiveness, sleeping problems, eating problems, lack of coordination (clumsiness), hyperactivity. One or more of these conditions are present in the group of children labeled minimal brain dysfunction (MBD). These children are often delayed in language development. The delay may be part of the MBD condition or because the condition causes behavior in which learning is very difficult or impossible.

Sharon is a difficult child to care for. She is always on the go. She is more than boisterous, she seems driven to constant activity. She has been diagnosed as "hyperactive." This activity is undirected. She picks up a toy for a minute, then drops it or, worse, throws it. Sometimes the toy hits someone or something. She is not trying to be destructive, she just never considers the consequences of what she does. At four years she should know enough to stay away from pots on the stove, but her mother must still watch that she doesn't knock them off and scald herself. Her speech is unclear and her sentences babyish for her age. Her vocabulary is poor, and she gets what she wants by pointing at it rather than asking for it by name. She is clumsy and often breaks toys that she is trying to play with. Chapter 3 has more information and advice for parents with children like Sharon.

Many children are troublesome and difficult to care for. How can you tell the difference between an active child who is always causing trouble, a "Dennis the Menace" but normal, and a child who is hyperactive? Clay, a neighbor of Sharon's, is also always getting into trouble. Clay's mother is driven to distraction by his capers which include attempting to wash books in the washing machine, painting the dog blue, picking up the telephone and dialing numbers. Clay is active but not hyperactive. His mischief is focused and purposeful. If he is motivated he can sit still. But Sharon cannot sit still long enough to listen to a story, an activity other children her age, including Clay, seem to enjoy. Sharon's disruptive behavior is almost involuntary—she cannot control it even if she wanted to.

Autism

Autism is the most extreme of the language disorders in children. Autism is a widely misunderstood condition which was thought to be emotionally based when it was first identified in the 1940s. An autistic child is a very strange individual who seems not to relate to or communicate with other people. The autistic child is likely not to speak at all. If such children do speak (usually in single words) it will not be to communicate. Their speech seems a solitary activity. Autistic children often pursue repetitious and other solitary activities such as rolling the same wheeled toy on the floor hours on end. The autistic child seems unaffectionate and has weird emotional responses such as laughing when there does not seem to be anything funny happening. For years this disorder was treated as if it were an emotional disturbance. Efforts at psychological remediation were dismal failures. It is more likely that autism is an impairment of the inborn capacity that children have to build their own language. The autistic child seems to understand very concrete things and be unable to deal with abstractions at all. Words are abstractions, symbols which stand for other things. If the autistic child does learn some words they are concrete and specific. The word *shirt* may stand for one particular shirt, but not all similar garments. Words that stand for intangibles such as *good* or *happy* are too abstract for a child with this disorder. Emotions are also abstractions, and this might explain why the autistic child looks like an emotionally disordered child. The child may feel emotions but not be able to understand them as such and not be able to react to them in any organized way. This unfortunate disorder illustrates how basic language is and how much of our functioning is determined by it. Chapter 3 discusses this condition more fully.

Combination of Problems

Although professionals divide speech problems into different categories, a given child may have more than one type of communication problem. For instance, a child with a bad articulation disorder or pronunciation problem can also have a language disorder problem along with it. In fact there are not many language disorders without speech sound problems. It is not always easy for a parent or teacher or speech clinician to understand the full extent of some communication problems. Often the clinician makes as educated a guess as possible about the nature of the problem, plans therapy based upon this guess and as the treatment goes on continually reevaluates. Sometimes one speech problem causes another. For instance if a child has a poor vocabulary because of a language problem, the hesitations and pauses while searching for words may sound like stuttering.[4] Once stuttering is perceived by the listener and conveyed to the child, genuine stuttering can begin. The person with cerebral palsy may have a language problem resulting from the same damage that caused the motor control difficulties or may be delayed in language development from the restricted environment caused by the motor difficulties. The child with a cleft palate may avoid moving certain portions of the speech apparatus because of pain from surgery. The avoidance of movements can lead to poor pronunciation habits. In this book I have simplified the cases as much as possible for the sake of clarity. But in real life communication problems are more complex.

There are many speculations on the causes of both the speech output problems—stuttering, pronunciation and voice—as well as the internal language problems. It is very difficult to figure out the exact causes in any given case. Undoubtedly some communication disorders can be prevented, but others cannot. The following chapters are meant to help you understand the communication difficul-

4. I remember a person who came to the speech clinic for stuttering. As we listened to the speech more carefully we heard sound formation problems overlaid on the stuttering. After a few sessions we realized that the language formation was not normal. Moreover, the voice was inappropriately soft and breathy. It was hard to know where to begin.

ties your child may be experiencing growing up and how you can help. But first you need to know what to expect from a normal child before you can consider if your child is not communicating normally.

Recognizing Speech Language and Hearing Problems

The following list is a rough guide of normal communication development. Many children develop on their own timetable without consulting lists such as this one. Some small children concentrate on other activities such as walking or climbing, leaving the talking for later. Although you know your child better than anyone else, this knowledge may make you less able to judge whether or not there is a communication problem. You can recognize a speech problem in a stranger immediately. But you are so used to the way your child speaks that you may not hear how different your child sounds. If a sympathetic friend or relative notices the way your child talks, there may be something wrong.

You may want professional help or you may want to work with your child yourself. Nevertheless the first step in helping your child is recognizing that there is a problem or that there might be a problem. The earlier that it can be recognized the better the chance that a handicapping condition can be avoided.

Normal Speech and Language Development[5]

0–6 Months
- Cries in many ways (from loud shrieks to soft whimpers, high and low pitched).
- Utters comfort sounds when feeling good (mmmmmm or aaaaaaah, etc.).
- Turns to sound of voices.
- Responds to tone of voice.
- Laughs, sometimes squeals.
- Jumps at sudden noise.
- Says syllables like "bee" and "moo" (they don't mean anything).
- Repeats syllables ("da da da da da").

5. *Mainstreaming Preschoolers* (Washington: U.S. Government Printing Office, 1978). Some of the communication development norms are taken from this series.

6–12 Months
- Imitates sounds parents make.
- Makes babbling sounds.
- Can be taught to clap hands and pat-a-cake.
- Understands "Bye-bye" and "Get up" if accompanied by gestures.
- Stops activity if parent says "No" sharply.
- Tries to imitate facial expressions.
- Plays peek-a-boo.

12–18 Months
- Says first words: "Mama," "Dada," maybe "kakuh" (cracker).
- Follows simple one-step directions such as "Come here."
- Can be understood by parents although most words do not sound perfect.
- Can point to some body parts when you name them, such as mouth, eye, hand, foot.
- Sometimes "parrots" your words.
- Turns toward speaker when name is called.
- Uses two or three word phrases such as "all gone" or "fall down" (although these sound like "aw gaw" or "faw dow").

18–24 Months
- Vocabulary goes from ten words to fifty in this time.
- Understands as many as three hundred words but does not speak them all.
- Says own name.
- Uses jargon or nonmeaningful "play speech."
- Asks "What's this?" often.

24–30 Months
- Joins in singing nursery rhymes with you, remembering most of the words.
- Can name a picture of any one of the following: bird, house, dog, baby.

30–36 Months
- Uses plurals.
- Can form sentences such as "Daddy came home."
- Has a vocabulary of nine hundred words.
- Can say most of the vowels: M, N, H, NG, F, W.[6]
- Shows the beginning of grammar: "No want eat" for "I don't want to eat."

6. J. E. Bernthal and N. W. Bankson. *Articulation Disorders* (Englewood Cliffs, NJ: Prentice-Hall, 1981). Different sound-acquisition ages come from a combination of surveys by M. Templin (1957), E. Poole (1934), B. Wellman (1931) and E. Prather with D. Hedrick and C. Kern (1975).

- Uses regular plurals and tense endings even on irregular verbs and nouns ("goed" for "went" and "mouses" for "mice").
- Uses negatives.
- Will give first and last name.
- Is understandable to sympathetic listener outside family.
- Refers to self as "I."
- Follows three-step directions in order such as, "Take off your coat, hang it up, go to the kitchen."

36–48 Months

- Has a vocabulary of 1500 words by four years.[7]
- Understands the concepts yesterday, today, tomorrow.
- Can speak all the vowel sounds.
- Can say Y, K, D, B, T, G.
- Can describe a picture.
- Knows some abstract words such as "tired" or "cold."
- Speaks in five-word sentences.
- Understands and expresses imaginary conditions such as "Let's pretend . . ." or "Suppose that . . ."
- Understands comparatives: "Which is bigger?"
- Shows occasional nonfluency, "I d-d-d-d-don't know."
- Knows age.
- Has speech intelligible to strangers although there are some noticeable sound mistakes.

48–60 Months

- Can describe what things are for: "A hat is to wear on your head."
- Knows the names of coins: penny, nickel, dime, quarter.[8]
- Can retell a story.
- Asks "why" questions and understands "because" answers.
- Understands sequencing of events.
- Has a vocabulary of 2200 words, which may include some you wish your child did not know or use.
- Can say R, S, SH, CH, J.
- Shows some normal nonfluency, especially when excited.
- Uses adult grammar, although a few incorrect forms may persist: "I don't want none."

7. N. Collins, G. Czuchna, G. Gill, G. O'Betts, and M. Stahl, *Teach Your Child to Talk* (New York: CEBCO Standard Publishing, 1969). This workshop manual is the source of the vocabulary size norms for the various ages.

8. I. L. Zimmerman, V. G. Steiner, and R. L. Evatt, *Preschool Language Scale* (Columbus: Charles E. Merrill, 1969). Picture identification and descriptions as well as certain observable language behaviors are from the norms on this general test of language development.

6 Years
- Can say L, TH, V and most consonant combinations (DR or ST etc.).
- Understands and uses the *wh* words (why, when, where, who, which, etc.).

7 Years
- Can say Z, ZH (televi*sion*) and TH as in *this*.
- Understands simple jokes.

School Years
- Learns to adjust speaking style to social situation (speaks differently on playground and to teacher).
- Grammar becomes more mature, can use longer complex sentences: "The boy who used to live next door called me."
- Appreciates puns and double meanings: "The turkey is ready to eat."

Danger Signals—Symptoms of Communication Problems

If your child really does have a speech, hearing or language problem, the earlier you know about it the sooner you can give your child the extra needed help. The following list shows some of the danger signals, conditions which may indicate your child has a communication problem.

0–6 Months
- Does not respond to the sound of others talking.
- Does not turn toward the speaker who is out of sight.
- Makes only crying sounds (no cooing or comfort sounds).

6–12 Months
- Does not babble (does not repeat syllables such as *guh guh guh* when alone).
- Does not discontinue activity upon your saying "no" sharply.

12–24 Months
- Does not say a meaningful word.
- Does not refer to self by name.
- Does not follow simple directions such as "Close the door."
- Vocabulary does not seem to increase.
- Does not talk at all at two years.

24–36 Months
- Does not say whole name (first and last names).
- Does not seem to understand *what* and *where* questions.

- Uses nonmeaningful gibberish (jargon) a great deal.
- Answers your question by repeating the question.
- Uses no more than one word at a time.
- Points to desired objects rather than naming them.
- Does not name any objects in pictures.

36–48 Months

- Leaves off the beginning consonants of words (*'ee* for *see*).
- Cannot be understood even by parents.
- Never uses sentences using subject-verb-object (Grandpa catches a fish).
- Does not use grammatic endings such as *-s* or *-ed.*
- Does not respond when you call name. Must be nudged to attend.
- Does not use two-to-three-word sentences.

48–60 Months

- Does not sequence events (mix the cake, then bake the cake, then eat the cake).
- Uses words only for concrete names of tangible things such as *dish* or *cookie*, never for abstract intangibles such as *hot, thirsty* or *pretty.*
- Cannot be understood by people outside the family.

5–6 Years

- Drops word endings.
- Does not show improvement in pronunciation problems.
- Uses poor word order ("Ball me not find," instead of "I don't find the ball").
- Cannot describe an outing or event.
- Exhibits habitual inattentiveness or dreaminess.

First Grade

- Stumbles over words and is aware of it.
- Needs to see speaker in order to listen.
- Uses grammatic forms in a very different way from the family's usage.
- Is reluctant to speak to new people.
- Has limited vocabulary compared to classmates.

All Ages

- Sounds very different from the speech of other children the same age.
- Shows frustration at not being understood much of the time. (Remember, however, a little frustration gives a child impetus to improve, but a lot of frustration is a sign of trouble.)
- Has trouble learning to read. (Reading problems may be based upon speech problems.)
- Has arithmetic difficulties. (Arithmetic requires a logic that needs

a developed grammar. Without this grammar, a child cannot handle math.)
- Does not seem to have friends at preschool or school.
- Develops sounds more than a year later than described above.
- Uses mostly vowel sounds.
- Has a voice that is monotone.
- Has a voice that is too loud or too soft.
- Has a voice pitched too high or low for the age and sex of the child.
- Has a voice that sounds husky or hoarse even when the child does not have a cold.
- Talks too fast to be clear.

3

How to Help Your
Language-Delayed Child

- *The Child Who Could Not Be Understood*
- *How Common Are Language Disabilities?*
- *What Does a Language-Disordered Child Sound Like?*
- *Does Your Child Have a Language Disorder?*
- *Language Disorders in a Mentally Retarded Child*
- *The Problem of Measuring Intellectual Capacity*
- *Learning Disabilities*
- *Different Points of View on Learning Disabilities*
- *How Common Are Learning Disabilities?*
- *Helping a Learning-Disabled Child*
- *An Aphasic Child*
- *The Child Who Seems Brain-Injured*
- *An Autistic Child*
- *Helping Your Child Build a Language*
- *Suggestions for the Parents of Language-Delayed Children*

The Child Who Could Not Be Understood

Nina looks like the ideal four-year-old. She plays happily by her-self, rides her tricycle around the yard and "helps" around the house, following simple directions. She has a sunny disposition and is the pet of her family and the neighbors. But she doesn't talk. It takes a while for a stranger to realize that she is not talking because she does say "Mama" and "Daddy" and "No." But the rest of her speech is incomprehensible gibberish. At first those unfamiliar with her assume that they cannot understand her pronunciation. Nina's mother thought for a while that her daughter actually was talking but that her pronunciation was too far "off" for her to understand. She would listen and listen to the gibberish and sometimes think she heard a word. But when she asked Nina to repeat it, the child couldn't or at least wouldn't do so. Friends and family tried to reassure the parents that Nina seemed so bright and responsive that there couldn't be anything to worry about; many children are slow in learning to talk clearly. This reassurance was repeated by Nina's pediatrician. The doctor saw a healthy, well-coordinated little girl with no physical problems and thought that time alone would clear up the speaking problem.

Nina's parents were worried. They had assumed that they could not understand what Nina was trying to say. But was she really saying anything? Was her gibberish any different from that of her eighteen-month-old cousin who was going through the play-speech stage of learning to talk? Could she be imitating talking without saying anything, the way she played at driving the car? Through pointing and grunting (with great expression) she managed to make her wants and needs known and did not suffer too much frustration. Nina was also helped in her communication by her two older sisters who were able to anticipate her needs before she had to express them.

Language and Speech

Nina's parents knew that hearing problems were a major cause in children failing to speak. Could Nina be deaf? They really could not believe she was because she always seemed to pay attention when her name was called. Moreover, Nina seemed to understand what other people were saying. If someone said that it was time to go out, Nina would get her coat. If asked to pick up her shoes, she would do so. But they did have Nina checked and, as they had expected, Nina's hearing was normal.

As the time for nursery school approached after her fourth birthday and only a few months remained until she would be placed in a group of children her age, her parents became aware of the difference between Nina's talking and that of other children. Could Nina be mentally retarded? Often retarded children are slow in learning to talk. They took Nina to a psychologist who specialized in measuring intelligence. The tests she was given measured two types of intellectual development, verbal and nonverbal. On the nonverbal tasks (such as putting the right shaped blocks into the right holes) Nina was as skilled as a normal child her age. On the verbal portion, however, Nina was a year and a half below her age. Nina was a four-year-old child with the verbal skills of a two-and-a-half-year-old. The psychologist told Nina's parents that she was not retarded but had a specific language delay.

Intellectual development is measured by observing two kinds of behavior: verbal (talking and understanding) and motor (athletic skills and manipulative ability). Nina's abilities in using her hands and body were normal for a four-year-old, but her verbal performance was behind schedule. As children like Nina grow up with impaired language ability, even the motor skills that had seemed all right at four years do not stay normal. The psychologist further explained that even arithmetic and geometry depend upon verbal thinking skills. Moreover, even such seemingly nonverbal activities as dancing and sports depend upon words in the conscious learning stage. It is possible to say that all learning is impeded by a lack of skill in language.

Nina's parents were concerned and a bit confused. They had thought there was something wrong with their child's speech and the psychologist kept talking about language. It was clear enough to them that the child was late in speaking, but why did the psychologist keep mentioning language? When they took Nina to a speech/language pathologist at the psychologist's suggestion, some of the confusion was cleared up. They learned that a person's speech is the verbal expression of that person's language. Some children speak but their speech is not clear; they know what they want to say but have difficulty in forming the words clearly. Other children like Nina do not speak because they have not learned the interior code that pairs words with things and events. No one could understand Nina's gibberish because her "language" had no real words at all.

The speech/language examination conducted by the pathologist was divided into two parts: comprehension and expression. The parents were not surprised that Nina was below her expected level in expression, nor were they surprised that her understanding was greater than her speech. But they were surprised to find that her understanding also fell below what was expected from a child of her age. It was true that she could point to some pictures correctly when words used to describe them were said, but she did not recognize as many objects as other four-year-olds. She missed grammatical meanings also, not only the difference between mother's cat and mother cat but the difference between girl and girls. The examiner's conclusion was that Nina, a bright and responsive little girl, was seriously delayed in developing her language as well as in developing her speech and should be given speech and language therapy.

Looking for a Cause

Although Nina's parents were reassured to find out that their child was not really mentally retarded nor was she deaf, why was she delayed in language? What was the cause of the delay? The speech/language clinician had asked Nina's mother many questions concerning her pregnancy and delivery and about Nina's medical and developmental history. Nina had run a high fever as a baby and had had a convulsion. At sixteen months she had fallen downstairs and had hit her head on a concrete sidewalk. Could one of these be the cause of her language delay? The clinician was reluctant to attribute the problem to any of these causes.[1] One or both of them could be the problem; any damage to the brain is suspect, but it would be impossible to say for sure. There are many children who have high fevers, convulsions and blows to the head who never have any language problems. There is no way of evaluating the suspect event to see if without it there would not have been a problem. Sometimes parents don't have any suspicious event to point to and yet their child is delayed in language. In these cases, speech clinicians are less interested in what caused the problem than in trying to remedy it.[2]

Although Nina was enrolled in speech and language therapy, Nina's parents realized that they still had a major part to play in helping Nina develop language. They both kept up with every-

1. R. C. Naremore, "Language Disorders in Children," from *Introduction to Communication Disorders* ed. by T. J. Hixon, L. D. Shriberg and J. H. Saxman (Englewood Cliffs, NJ: Prentice-Hall, 1980). It is not really useful to search for the cause of the language disability because the cause is probably irreversible in most cases. It is more useful to concentrate on measuring the actual behavior—what Nina can and cannot do.

2. F. R. Kleffner, *Language Disorders in Children* (Indianapolis: Bobbs-Merrill Educational Publishing Co., 1978). "A language disorder produces effects which will tend to perpetuate its existence." Thus looking for the cause may be impossible because it is a multi-leveled history of causes.

thing that Nina was doing and learning in the clinic and with help from the clinician tried to reinforce at home the new things that Nina learned in therapy. They also tried to create a favorable climate at home for Nina's speaking, learning new ways to help Nina increase her understanding.

Giving the Language-Delayed Child a Chance to Speak and to Understand

The first way Nina's parents changed things at home was to get the older girls to stop "reading" Nina's mind and doing her talking for her. The girls had been motivated by love and a desire to help. The parents, realizing this, enlisted the sisters' help a different way: by letting Nina do her own talking. Both the parents and the sisters also had to stop worrying about and correcting Nina's pronunciation. With these things in mind, the family developed a pattern of dealing with Nina's nonverbal communication. When Nina would point at what she wanted, accompanied by one of her plaintive grunts, the family would not respond right away. If they thought that the word was one that Nina had learned, they would wait to give her a chance to say it. If she still did not attempt the word they would repeat it several times, then wait and give her another chance to say it. This usually worked to get Nina to try the word. Even if it did not, however, Nina had a chance to hear the word several times.

Nina's parents realized that they had not given Nina a chance to understand them. The speech clinician advised keeping sentences down to no more than four words when talking to Nina in order to simplify the task of understanding. Her parents had been overloading Nina by expecting her to comprehend too many words in too short a time. She had understood some of them but not all.

One thing that Nina did that was upsetting and annoying to her parents was "parroting" back what they had just said to her. They came to understand, in time, that this was Nina's way of holding what she had just heard in her mind long enough for her to decode the message. It not only prolonged the talk, but the repetition (echolalia) stopped the speaker from saying anything new to add more confusion. Of course Nina did not work out this strategy consciously.

Learning How to Elicit a Response

Nina's family found that it helped if they gave her extra time to respond. They also came to understand that direct questions that can be answered "yes" or "no" or by nodding or shaking the head actually inhibit talk. They had thought that they were having a communicative talk with Nina, but actually *they* were doing all the talking. Nina's parents noticed that certain relatives would think that Nina was talking in a conversation like the following:

> WELL-MEANING RELATIVE: Do you like school?
> NINA [nodding head]: Mmm-hmmm.
> WMR: Do you go to nursery school?
> NINA: Uh-huh.
> WMR: Do you play with blocks?
> NINA: Uh-huh.
> WMR: Do you like TV?
> NINA [nodding]: Uh.
> WMR: I bet you like *Sesame Street*.
> NINA: Uh-huh [nodding].
> WMR: Looking forward to Santa Claus?
> NINA: Mmmm.
> WMR [to Nina's mother]: Such a sweet little girl. We're having such a nice talk.
> NINA'S MOTHER [smiling, nodding]: Mmm-hmmm.

Nina did not say a word. Nina did not have to understand a word that the relative was saying. There may not have been any communication whatsoever, and yet the relative thought that Nina was talking. An occasional relative who makes this type of mistake will not cause any harm, but if this is the customary style of speech situations at home, there is no impetus or need for Nina to try to talk.

Her parents found that Nina could be encouraged to try to talk if they would ask her, when she showed them a picture she had painted, "Tell me about this," rather than "Is this a picture of a house?" In the first question Nina is encouraged to find the words to explain her picture. The exchange can be expanded and elaborated as the parent points to various parts of the picture stimulating more talk. With the second question the conversation can be finished with one word.

Building a Vocabulary

Nina and her parents found that speech therapy was very much like nursery school but more structured. A game similar to follow-the-leader would begin by Nina's following her leader by moving her arms and then her head in different ways. Then she would follow her leader by moving her mouth in certain ways and then making noises after her leader like *moo, baw* and *bee*. Somehow the noises changed and *moo* became *moon* and *baw* became *ball* and so forth. The objective of the therapy was to break language learning into small steps so that the child's capacity to learn language would have a chance.

Because Nina's parents knew what was going on in the clinic they were able to reinforce the subjects that Nina had learned. When Nina had learned the difference between *in, under, around, beside* and *over,* they could expect her to know these words at home. She could then be asked "Bring me the shoes under the bed." In order to build a vocabulary, the clinician introduced words in groups so that the new words would be classified. One group might be means of transportation (cars, trains, airplanes, etc.); another would be household appliances (washing machines, refrigerators etc.), a third would be clothing. The clinician starts with pairing the word with the object itself, if possible, or a toy representation of the object (toy car) or a picture of the object. Once the names and functions are mastered, the clinician can describe characteristics of the objects. For example, an airplane is something you ride in, a way to go places. Then its abstract qualities can be discussed; that is, it is big, loud and very fast. When several vocabulary units have been mastered Nina will be ready to move into more abstract ideas such as things that are big (elephants, trucks, buildings) and things that are small (pins, seeds).

Guided by the activity in the clinic the parents were able to continue the subject at home. When the subject was transportation, Nina's mother pointed out the real trucks and cars on the road on the trip home. Later Nina's father showed Nina pictures of trains and airplanes from a magazine. Not only was Nina able to continue learning about these things outside the clinic, but was able to see real examples of the words she had learned. If in the clinic she had learned to pair the word *truck* with only a picture of a truck, her concept of the word *truck* would be limited. The word and the idea of truck are better mastered when the sound of the word conjures up in her mind the actual truck on the highway as well as the picture she saw in the clinic. Nina's parents realized that it was up to them to help her use what she had learned in therapy in the outside world. We have found in working with language-delayed children that children of parents who make an effort to support what is going on in the clinic progress better than those who do not.

It may surprise parents that supposedly simple concrete words such as *dress* exist in an elaborate network of personal meanings and functions. For example, a dress is more than an article of clothing. It (1) is worn by girls not boys, (2) must cover the upper body as well as have a skirt (not be just a skirt or a blouse), (3) can be any color, (4) includes the present Nina got for her birthday (a yellow dress), (5) is the garment she and other girls wear to church (never pants or shorts), (6) is never worn to picnics (always pants or shorts). A possible conversation might be:

NINA: Nina dress [pointing to own dress].
MOTHER: Yes, this is Nina's dress.
NINA: Daddy dress [points to father's shirt].
MOTHER: No—not a dress [shakes head].
NINA: Daddy wear____
MOTHER: Yes, Daddy wears a shirt and pants—not a dress.
NINA: Mommy dress [points to mother's dress].
MOTHER: Yes, Mommy and Nina wear dresses.

It is up to Nina's family to help her develop this elaborate network around simple-seeming words. Every concrete thing has a name, a purpose, is made of something, has a particular appearance, is a member of a class of things (in this case clothing), is used by certain people, is used at certain times. How much richer and more informative this is for Nina than merely identifying a picture by a name.

How Common Are Language Disabilities?

The incidence of children failing to acquire any language at all is .6 percent (six out of a thousand) in children under four years. Many of these children seem to learn some language when they get older because the incidence drops to .08 percent of children aged four to seventeen. This means that eight out of 10,000 children ages four to seventeen have no oral language at all. Delayed language learning, however, is more common. About 6 percent of children have some language delay. Add to this acquired language disabilities and you get a total of 6.5 percent of children in the school years who have a language disorder.[3] Not included in these figures are the children who have nonpathological language problems arising from foreign birth and bilingualism. Because there is now more consciousness of schoolchildren with language problems, we are seeing an increase in its prevalence.

What Does a Language-Disordered Child Sound Like?

The most obvious sign of a language disorder is muteness. That is rare, however; the usual speech of a language-disabled child is peculiar speech. It may sound like the speech of a younger child, as was the case with Nina. There are, however, clues to language disability in the type of utterance a child makes.

There are problems in putting words together to say what the child wants them to mean. "Daddy car drive" said by a four-year-old child or older instead of "Daddy drives the car" would mean that the child has not mastered word order. Sometimes there is grammatic confusion such as "Billy play room" instead of "Billy plays in the room." Notice also that these examples did not have the regular grammatic endings—no final s's. Sometimes the language-disabled child has a poor vocabulary and tries to make up for the lack of words by circumlocutions such as "thing you eat with" instead of fork. Sometimes the child uses indefinite words like "junk" or "stuff" in place of definite nouns. Of course all children use these words to some extent, but the language-disordered child would use them noticeably more frequently than a normal child.

3. C. Van Riper, *Speech Correction: Principles and Practice* (Englewood Cliffs, NJ: Prentice-Hall, 1978). The incidence of language disabilities are from a 1972 survey. However, E. Wiig, in *Human Communication Disorders: An Introduction* (Columbus: Charles E. Merrill, 1982), says that the estimates of learning disabilities in schoolchildren range from 1 to 30 percent and the prevalence of language disorders among the learning disabled ranges from 40 to 60 percent. This would work out to a range of 0.4 to 18 percent of *all* schoolchildren with language disorders.

Does Your Child Have a Language Disorder?

How can you tell if your child has a language disorder? Even the most observant and careful parents can be astonished to find that their child has a language disorder. The condition is by no means obvious. By comparison, it is relatively easy to spot a speech disorder. We are all quite sensitive to small variations in speaking. Though we may not be able to tell precisely what is wrong with a person's speech, we do recognize poor speech when we hear it. Speech is an outward behavior: It shows. Language refers to an interior structure which we can only guess at on the basis of what we hear from the outside. Since most language problems include speech problems, the speech problem is apparent but the language problem may be overlooked. Language development is subtle. Do not be surprised if you cannot immediately uncover a language problem in your child. But if you do suspect such a problem, refer to the guidelines and danger signals in speech development summarized in Chapter 2.

Certain conditions might predispose your child to language difficulty. A difficult pregnancy and birth may have damaged the baby so that the language learning centers are not right. This does not mean, though, that every baby who has a bad prenatal and delivery history will be language impaired. If your child has had high fevers and/or convulsions there is a possibility of some brain damage. Again, not every child who has had high fevers and convulsions is language impaired, but the child is in a higher-risk category. There are probably many instances of babies undergoing brain damage early in their lives without apparent permanent harm. The child simply develops using undamaged portions of the brain.

Any incident or illness in which the brain is starved of oxygen also puts the child in a higher-risk category, such as an accidental blow to the head or a poisoning (see Janet later in this chapter). Hearing loss is another cause for children not to develop language normally. Chapter 4 explains about the problems of deaf and hard-of-hearing children. There are congenital handicapping conditions which may be or are always accompanied by language problems. Cerebral palsy (Chapter 7) does not inevitably result in a language disorder, but it is a possibility. Cleft lip and cleft palate (Chapter

6) can have language delay as well as the speech problems brought on by the structural differences. Many conditions or syndromes (collections of symptoms) include some degree of mental retardation. Mental retardation can also exist without any other handicaps. Any case of mental retardation is going to mean some degree of language disability. Retarded people have difficulty learning, and one of the things they have difficulty learning is language. The language level they achieve depends upon the degree of the retardation. Often they can talk but their language is limited.[4]

Language Disorders in a Mentally Retarded Child

Karl was born with Down's syndrome, a condition in which there is an extra chromosome in the cells. The doctor at Karl's delivery saw the peculiar lower eyelid, a single crease on the palm of the hand and a generally flaccid muscle tone, all symptoms of Down's. The appearance of the lower eyelid gave the baby a faintly Oriental look, which accounts for its former and now disfavored name, Mongolism or Mongoloid idiocy. Accompanying these physical characteristics is mental retardation. The physician was discouraging and when he broke the news to Karl's parents advised them to put the child in an institution. They had looked forward to this baby so much that at first they could not believe such dreadful news. They decided against putting Karl in an institution. During the next few months Karl's parents went through a period of mourning in which they buried the baby of their dreams and learned to accept the baby they actually had. They were lucky in finding a support group in the local chapter of the Association for Retarded Citizens. They learned that although Down's syndrome always means mental retardation, there are greater or lesser degrees of mental retardation. They found out from the ARC that Down's children are usually not severely retarded; that is, unable to take care of their physical needs; some, in fact, function almost at the normal level. They knew from the very beginning that there would be problems for Karl in learning and developing language, but they learned that a retarded person does learn although not so

4. R. D. Hubbell, *Children's Language Disorders: An Integrated Approach* (Englewood Cliffs, NJ: Prentice-Hall, 1981). Hubbell points out that there is not a strict linear cause-and-effect relationship between environmental events and the language difficulty but rather a transactional relationship between environmental and constitutional causes, each affecting the other. This is similar to Kleffner (op. cit.).

rapidly, and has formative language learning times as do normal children.[5] Karl's parents were able to utilize this early learning time. Instead of waiting to see how far Karl would develop on his own, they became active in bringing more stimulation to him, giving him more opportunities to learn to make up for his difficulty in learning.

Compensatory Stimulation

Karl's parents understood that the main difference between children of normal intelligence and children like Karl, who had some degree of intellectual impairment, was that normal children "pick things up" while retarded children have to be taught. Other than being provided with a healthy emotional and stimulating intellectual environment, normal children do not need to be consciously taught in the early years. They learn things on their own: talking, walking, climbing, getting into things, tastes, textures, sights and so forth. But for Karl, it would not be enough simply to talk in Karl's presence for him to pick up words and their meanings. Karl's mother and father needed to direct words toward Karl, demonstrating their meanings at the same time. For example, when putting on Karl's socks and shoes, Karl's father would say "Here's a shoe shoe shoe," while holding up the shoe. Then "put on foot foot foot" while holding Karl's foot. Then he would do the same thing with the other foot. These lessons would have to be repeated many times. This may sound tiresome, but Karl's parents found that the one thing they did not have to teach Karl was affection. He turned out to be a very affectionate baby and was eager to please his parents. When just a few months old Karl was already a willing and motivated "student." At six months of age Karl's parents worked with him. They imitated his syllables over and over so that he got the extra stimulation of simple speech sounds. They brought him noisemakers of all kinds so that he could listen to many different sounds. Knowing that the sense of touch is

5. B. B. Schlanger, *Mental Retardation* (Indianapolis: Bobbs-Merrill Co., 1976). Estimates of speech and language problems among the mentally retarded: less than half for the mildly retarded (IQ 50–70, 2.6 percent of the total population); 90 percent for moderate to severe MR (IQ 20–49, 0.3 percent of the total population) and all profoundly MR (IQ less than 20 or 0.1 percent of the total population). These statistics were gathered from institutionalized patients who tend to have lower language and speech functioning than those in homes.

very important to babies, they brought him things with different textures, things that were rough or smooth or hard, soft, warm or cold. They talked about these textures before he could understand, but kept what they said very simple so that he would have an easier time when he did begin to understand. Because the Down's child often has weakened muscles, they helped Karl exercise. As Karl's father manipulated the baby's legs and feet, he would name the part of the body being moved so that Karl exercised not only his limbs but his listening skills. What Karl's parents did with Karl was no different from what parents did with normal babies; they just did it more often.

Karl's parents group discussed the unique contemporary position in history of Down's children. Although the condition has probably always occurred, in the past people gave up trying to teach such children. The belief was that it was useless to try to teach anything to children who had trouble learning. The philosophy has turned around in the present generation. Now the idea is that if a child has trouble learning, you have to teach harder to compensate. The result is that children with this condition function at levels that surprise their parents and especially the doctors. Limits of intellectual development cannot be determined from looking at adults with Down's. They probably did not have the special education that such children have now. Karl's parents prefer not to think about the ultimate limits of their son's skills but instead strive for some progress at every stage of his childhood.

Karl was able to learn words but not at the same time as normal children. His language development was not very different from normal, but it took much longer, as did Karl's physical development. He did not sit unaided alone until he was eighteen months old (the normal age is about six months). He was three years old before he walked—and only after a great deal of training. Karl is not as mobile as most babies and so is easier to live with because he is not always getting into things. Karl's slower language development is part of the overall developmental delay, but it is possible that some of his lack of vocabulary is because he is confined by his own motor difficulties and has less need for new words. Just as the physical exploration that most children go through may enhance language exploration, the lack of physical exploration may inhibit it.

Gestures as a Communication Aid

Karl said his first word at about age three, and by four his vocabulary had reached fifty words (compared to about 1500 words for a normal child). The words he says are difficult to understand. Karl's tongue is broad and flat and does not seem to move as easily as normal tongues do. Karl's parents see progress in his development, but it is obvious that with such a gap it is unlikely he will ever catch up with normal children. They do not expect him to grow up to be a nuclear scientist, a lawyer or a businessman, but they have faith that he will learn to communicate.

Karl was enrolled in a special preschool program. It was thought that if gestures were combined with the spoken word, children like Karl could learn words more easily. Karl's parents had found out on their own that gestures paired with words were easier for Karl to understand. Words are over so quickly that it is hard for a person whose mind works slowly to comprehend them, while a gesture can be held longer. His parents were afraid, however, that if they used gestures too often Karl might prefer them to the spoken word and communicate only in sign language which neither they nor their family could understand. But they discovered that the gestures learned in school did not replace the spoken word at all. The school used a simplified version of American Sign Language (one of the manual languages used by the deaf), and Karl would demonstrate his new words using the speech and the sign at the same time. The signs worked as a mnemonic or memory aid for Karl, and so instead of it being more difficult to learn two forms of communication, it seemed easier.

While Karl was receiving special preschool education in a language and development program, his parents tried to widen his world and experiences. They took him to picnics, the zoo, carnivals, the circus and the beach. They exposed him to normal children, not for him to compete with but to serve as models for him. They were eager to give him a wide variety of social experiences.

All too often children with Down's syndrome as well as other mentally retarded children become overweight. One explanation for this may be because such children do not know when they are full and so continue eating. Or it may be that because they are physically inactive they do not need as much food as other children. Another explanation may be that mealtime is a time when the whole family sits down together as equals. Karl can eat as well as anybody and does so, perhaps excessively, because the sensation and satisfaction of eating is the same for everybody no matter what their IQ and Karl enjoys his "normalcy." His parents try to provide social activities in which he can participate other than eating. Karl's father took him fishing and to everyone's delight the fishes were biting Karl's line. Of course these activities are opportunities to use whatever communication skills he has learned.

The Problem of Measuring Intellectual Capacity

In most cases where there are no physical symptoms to alert parents to the possibility of a mental retardation problem, valuable time is lost before they realize the child is not developing on time. Therefore the sooner parents discover retardation in their child the earlier they will be able to give special help. Karl's parents had the advantage of knowing Karl would be intellectually limited from the beginning. For most children, however, without physical symptoms indicating retardation, intellectual testing would be the only way to find out. But early testing in children is unreliable. Because it is impossible to measure intellectual capacity directly, it is inferred by a child's performance on an IQ test. The individual's performance is then compared to the average performance on this same test of many children of the same age as the test taker (normal performance). And if the individual child's score falls a specified amount lower than normal, the child is classified as being retarded; that is, the child's learning is slower than normal, the test indicating how much the child has learned. The problem in this kind of test is that not every child has been exposed to the same learning experiences; the test tests what has been learned or not learned, not why it was not learned. And because one particular performance at a particular time is being evaluated, there may be other reasons for a child not performing well on a test, and therefore being labeled as retarded when actually the child is normal. But just as there are factors that can depress IQ results, there are factors that can increase them. It makes no sense to say that a person can perform beyond competence, but a performance can come close to the maximum level for that person. It is unlikely that Karl's parents could really raise his innate mental capacity by their program of stimulation and education, but they could increase his level of functioning. They learned what parents of all children (retarded or not) should know: that they can increase what the child does in fact learn. Moreover it may be true that Karl's parents did to some extent increase his capacity to learn by helping him acquire the most important tool in learning—language. Language is the memory storage system and without it there would be no way to hold on to what has been learned.

If you compare Nina with Karl or other children like them, there is a difference that would not be obvious in their communication development. When Karl was given two types of intellectual tasks, verbal and nonverbal, he showed delayed development in both. His language delay was part of total delay. Nina, on the other hand, showed normal development in the nonlanguage tasks which contrasted with her poor showing on language ability. This difference in abilities showed that Nina had a specific language delay, so her therapy was directed at this one aspect of development. Karl, on the other hand, needed a more varied approach to help him with all kinds of learning. Sometimes children have very specific problems in their learning which can "hang up" their whole development.

Learning Disabilities

Language Disorders and a Problem of Visual Orientation

A child may have problems in spatial orientation; that is, perceiving the placement of things in space and remembering where they are. The ability to place things in space is learned. Observant parents can see their crawling baby intently examining the underside of a chair, then climbing on top of the chair, then later studying it from the sides and back. In this way the different views of the chair are integrated into the whole three-dimensional object. If for some reason a child did not learn to integrate the many visual sensations possible from looking at a single object, the pairing of a word to that object might be difficult or impossible. To such a child the world would be a confusing and unpredictable place. Everything the child looked at would be new and unknown. Most parents cannot notice a problem such as this in their child during the early years. They might notice that their child had fewer words or that his behavior was not well organized, but often they would not know of any real difficulty until the child entered school, where his perceptual problem would impact directly on the academic demands of reading and writing. This may show up in reading problems, in which the exact position of the letters in relation to each other is very important as well as the discrimination between similar letters (*b* and *d* for instance).

Helping your child understand the physical environment. If they could have suspected a visual learning disability in the early years, parents could have helped by leading the child to learn through other senses. For instance if the child were having difficulty recognizing that the view from the back of the chair and the view from the side of the chair were still views of the same object, the parents could have encouraged the child to touch the chair. As the child experiences the chair through hands and fingers the parent talks about the chair. As the child reaches around the seat from the back the parent says "You can't see that part from here but it is still there." This is followed up later with games that exercise the child's visual perception. A picture of a car on a street with the roof of the car against the pavement and the wheels in the air is shown to the child. "What's wrong with this?" the parent asks. If the child cannot figure it out the parent gets a toy car (one with rollable wheels), puts it on the floor upside down and says to the child, "Make it go." If the child still does not fix it so the car can roll, the parent demonstrates, saying that the wheels have to touch the ground to make the car roll. The child could then roll the car several times while the parent reinforces the action with words by saying "Roll the car on the ground." Then the parent goes back to the more difficult picture of the upside-down car.

How do these activities and others similar to them help a child with a visual perceptual problem? In a sense the hands are being used to build the mental picture that the child's eyes were unable to build. This mental picture is necessary in learning language, especially names of things. The mental picture most people have of nouns allows for all the possible variations of the noun. For instance, when you hear the word "dog" there is an image in your mind of a moderate-size animal with four legs, long nose and fur. It may be a particular dog you know, but your image is elastic enough to admit a tiny chihuahua or a collie into the idea of dog. If your mental picture were not so elastic you would have to have a special word for each type of dog—not only every breed but every mutt. You help your child form an elastic mental picture of a chair by showing the characteristics of "chairness" which are there regardless of the particular view or of the particular chair. With the car game the parent is trying to help the child learn about the physical relationships of objects to their environment. The car is an object which works in only one position—wheels on the pavement. The understanding of this gained through the concrete situation—using the toy car—can then help the child understand the problem in the less concrete situation of the picture. When the parent teaching the child runs into a task the child cannot do, the parent backs off and switches to a simpler task until the child can do it. This is an important technique. In general a child can understand a real object more readily than a picture of that object, and can understand a picture of the object more easily than the spoken word for that object. A child is also more likely to understand what you want if you demonstrate the action first; then you and the child do it together, and finally the child does it alone.

You do not have to wait for your child to exhibit problems in order to play these games. Any two-year-old could play the game with the chair, maybe even an eighteen-month-old. Any three-year-old would enjoy the car game. It could be that experiencing these objects is enough to teach children about the relationship of objects to each other. But some children may need the more organized presentation of these experiences that such games provide.

Figure-Ground Discrimination

Confusion about where things are is only one "hang up" a child can encounter. Some children have problems focusing on one specific sound or conversation while ignoring the background sensation. In general you can pay attention to a conversation even though there is street noise outside the window. You have learned not to hear what you are not interested in listening to while being carefully attentive to what you do want to hear. You also look at what you want to focus on and don't see things in the background. This is called figure-ground discrimination. In all probability you were not born with this skill—you had to learn it. Some children do not seem to learn it at the time that other children do. They cannot ignore the background noise around them. There is too much coming in through their eyes and ears for them to cope with.

Sometimes children with figure-ground discrimination problems do focus on one object in their sensory environment but not the same one as most people do. Small children who are developing normally often notice things that the rest of us ignore, being distracted by a blemish or imperfection while not paying attention to the object. This is known by magicians who do sleight-of-hand tricks which depend upon distracting the audience so that the real movement is not seen. Small children often will not be distracted by the "show" and keep staring at the "business end" of the performance and never experience the illusion. They have not learned to look at what they are supposed to look at.

By age four and five a child should be as easy to fool as an adult. The child should pay attention to that part of the total sensation which carried the most meaning. The child should be able to hear the spoken message through the noise (meaningless sound). Because it is necessary at all stages in learning language to pick out what is meaningful and to disregard what is nonmeaningful, problems of figure-ground discrimination will have an adverse effect on a child's communication development. The infant in the second half year of life is busy learning to distinguish the parts of the speech signal (including the tone of voice) that say something from the parts of the speech signal that don't. Later, at the time of learning to understand, it is necessary for the child to listen for the words that are already known.

Many learning disabled children seem to have very short attention spans or have difficulty paying attention to anything. If a child is unable to pick out one thing to concentrate on out of the many sensations coming in, such behavior is not surprising.

Sequencing

Sometimes children have trouble sequencing events or things, remembering the order of what they heard or saw. This is related to the problem of spatial orientation mentioned earlier, but it can also include temporal (time) orientation. A child who has trouble sequencing the order of things heard may say "shoe red" instead of "red shoe" or misorder the sounds within the words, making speech unintelligible. Word meanings become confused to the temporally disoriented child, who may say "last" when "first" is what is meant: "Me last" instead of "I'm first."

Different Points of View on Learning Disabilities

Since discovering that children could have specific learning problems that account for slow personal or academic development, there has been an effort to classify these disabilities.[6] The different ways to do so depend on your point of view: legal, psychological or behavioral.

PL-94-142 is a federal law which states that every child who is disabled is entitled to the appropriate compensatory education for that child to reach full potential. The learning disabled therefore have a legal classification based upon the academic difficulties they present. These include problems in oral expression, listening comprehension, basic reading skill, reading comprehension, written expression, mathematics calculation and mathematics reasoning. All these areas involve language skills with the possible exception of mathematics calculation. A child with any of these specific problems is classified in the special population under the law.

The teacher or the psychologist is not so interested in the legal classifications as in the learning process which is impaired. It is necessary to understand what is wrong or atypical in the child's learning process to design a program to overcome it. Here the categories are: auditory or visual learning disabilities (difficulty in receiving information through the eyes and ears and making sense of it), sensory-motor problems (difficulty in relating what you see or hear with the movements you are making), memory problems and perceptual handicaps. Often the child will have more than one of these problems.

The behavioral classifications are of greater interest to parents because they describe what the parent and the child have to cope with in an everyday situation. Usually children exhibit more than one of these behaviors, and any one of them is a deterrent to learning. They are: hyperactivity (need to move constantly), impulsivity (acting without thinking of the consequences), clumsiness, perseveration (the repetition of an action or an utterance over

6. B. B. Osman, *Learning Disabilities: A Family Affair* (New York: Warner Books, 1980). The U.S. Office of Education defines learning disabilities to include problems in listening, thinking, reading, writing, spelling and arithmetic that are not due to mental retardation, emotional disturbance or environmental disadvantage. The author notes that it is not easy to make this distinction in actual cases.

and over) and distractability (inability to concentrate or pay attention).[7]

How Common Are Learning Disabilities?

As in trying to figure out the prevalence of language disorders,
there are widely differing estimates of the incidence of learning
disabilities. It is quite possible that the surveys include children
with language disorders who are counted as having learning disabilities and vice versa. The estimates in the past have fluctuated
from 1 to 30 percent of schoolchildren.[8] The high figures are suspect especially if there is an allocation of funds involved. In a
period of budget cuts, the admitted incidence figures will probably be low so that limited funds can serve fewer children and the
school can still comply with the law. There is always some discre-
tion in where you set the borderline between boisterous and hyperactive or auditory perceptual disability and poor listening habits. A
reasonable estimate of the prevalence in 1980 is that fewer than 1
percent of children are profoundly learning disabled (these may be
also counted in other handicap populations). Three to 4 percent of
schoolchildren have moderate learning disabilities, and 10 to 15
percent have mild learning disabilities. The last group may get
along on their own, making up the bottom of a regular class in
school. For the children with moderate learning disabilities, special
education may be the difference between their being able to function as normal adults and being handicapped all their lives.

Helping a Learning Disabled Child

Morris is a child whose world is a chaos to him. Not only does he
have trouble remembering the order of the words he hears but he
has trouble remembering when things are supposed to happen.
Suppertime often comes as a surprise to him. His spatial confusion
is sometimes so bad that he loses his way around the house. Morris

7. R. J. Van Hattum, *Communication Disorders: An Introduction* (New York:
Macmillan Publishing Co., 1980). The different points of view of learning disabilities
classification.

8. E. Wiig, "Language Disabilities in the School Age Child," from *Human Communication Disorders: An Introduction* (Columbus: Charles E. Merrill Publishing Co.,
1982). That 1 to 30 percent range in the estimate of learning disabilities in schoolchildren
shows how difficult it is to make sense of prevalence figures.

was slow in learning to talk, and when he did start talking no one could understand him. He tended to simplify words, using only one consonant for every consonant in the word; thus *dog* became *gog* and *tomato* became *tato* which also stood for *potato*. When he reached the stage at which other children begin to use grammatic endings he would use the ending-*ing* on everything. His pronouns were confused. He would say *you* when he meant *me* and *me* when he meant *you*. Even if you could understand the words Morris was attempting to say you would be confused at the message. "Wanting you going no" could be interpreted as "Yes, I want to go." In Morris's topsy-turvy world *up* was *down*, *in* was *out*, *yes* was sometimes *no* and *last* was *first*. Morris's mistakes were not the usual mistakes children make as they are growing up—they were bizarre. Nina had a specific delay in her development of language while the other aspects of her development were normal; her language did come in the normal way, just on a different timetable. Karl, too, had normal development but just not in the normal time. No one could recognize the speech of a younger child in Morris.

Most children develop their language and speech along a certain pattern, a certain order. They may go through these "stages" fast or slowly. But Morris followed a different plan or pattern in his learning. His mistakes were not like the speech mistakes other children made. His language was not so much immature as unique; for instance, *yes* and *no* are not ordinarily confused by children at any age old enough to know the words, but Morris did confuse them.

It may be that Morris will eventually develop some skill in communication, going through processes and stages that are unique to him. It may be, too, that he will eventually function as a normal adult. Adults have the advantage of having more control over their environments than children. If reading and arithmetic are difficult for him he will be able to arrange his adult life to avoid them. Adults with learning disabilities can avoid those areas they cannot operate in. But first Morris has to grow up. School is arranged to present certain material in certain ways at certain ages of a child's life. He will need help to get the necessary basic schooling. Morris may be diagnosed as dyslexic when he gets to school (dyslexia means a specific language disability in reading), because his reading problems will be due to his difficulties in learning the language he is supposed to read. Morris's "dyslexia" may merely be that he is not yet ready to learn to read at the age other children learn. There is some debate on whether a child like Morris should be considered language-deficient or language-different. There is some evidence that children like Morris can grow out of the problem. Their development is different from normal and examined while in progress seems slow, bizarre, deficient. But the final proficiency will be normal even if arrived at by a different route.

Morris's parents want to do something to help him, not simply hope he will grow out of his problem. Suppose that he doesn't grow out of his strange speech? Suppose that when he's eight years old, his parents come to the conclusion that he will not develop a normal language without special help? He will have lost some valuable learning time between the ages of three (when the problem was first noticed) and eight. He will have also suffered emotionally. Being confused and unable to communicate to others or form one's own thoughts clearly leads to unhappiness and poor adjustment. By eight years old, Morris would feel himself a failure in many areas. Therefore Morris's parents want to get started as soon as possible. They want special training for Morris and need to supplement it with more than the usual help at home.

The speech clinician and special preschool teacher worked with Morris's parents on various things they could do at home. When they wanted to explain something to Morris they did so with as few words as possible, speaking slowly and clearly. If appropriate, the parent can accompany direction with a gesture or physically move the child through the motion. Morris's father taught him to throw a ball by holding Morris's hand while his hand was holding the ball and physically putting Morris's arm and hand through the motions. Being a patient man, he realized that Morris would need a great deal of practice to perfect ball throwing.

Morris was having trouble dressing himself. It was hard enough figuring out which limbs belonged in which holes in the clothing, but when the clothes were all collapsed in a pile it was very difficult for Morris to find the sleeves at all, let alone the right sleeve for the right arm and the left sleeve for the left arm. Morris's mother broke down the task of putting on a shirt into tiny steps. She started by putting the shirt flat on the table with the label down and the bottom toward Morris. Morris then put both arms in the tube of the shirt from the bottom. The next step was to find the armholes with the hands that were inside the shirt. Then put the hands through the armholes. Now raise the arms so that the shirt was above Morris's head. Then push the head through the bottom of the shirt. Put the neck hole over the head. Then pull from the underarms to settle the shirt on the shoulders and finally Morris was to pull the shirt bottom down to his waist. Morris's mother did not simply tell Morris these eight steps. She described each step as she put on the T shirt, showing, doing and talking (using the same words each time). Then when the procedure became a ritual, she helped Morris with the first seven steps, letting him do the last step unassisted. When he was finished with his one step the shirt was on. Then Morris's mother let him do the last two steps. She increased the number of steps for Morris bit by bit (last three then last four etc.) until Morris did the whole thing on his own.[9]

Morris's parents also learned that consistency was more important for their child than with most children. His father decided that Morris should hang up his coat on a hook every time he came in from the outside. He then saw to it that the coat was indeed hung up every time. If Morris came in and dumped his coat on the floor, Morris's father would call him back and by spoken direction accompanied by gesture remind Morris to pick up his coat.

At first Morris's parents were not sure that teaching him the skills of dressing himself and neatness was a way to help him with his language. But they came to realize after a while that language applies to the child's whole world and whole experience. By helping him master a previously incomprehensible task such as putting on a shirt, they were helping him make sense out of things that were difficult at first. One of the tools used in learning to put on a shirt was language. Not only did language facilitate putting on the shirt, but putting on the shirt reinforced language. Moreover, a child like Morris is not always able to keep track of all the parts of his body. Putting on the shirt forces him to deal with his own body parts. In addition, the act of putting on a shirt broken down into small steps helps Morris put things in the proper order. It is physically impossible for Morris to go through the putting on of a shirt in any other sequence. It is possible to speak in any order but only one order will be understood. When Morris's parents saw that they

9. *Mainstreaming Preschoolers: Children with Learning Disabilities* (Washington: U.S. Government Printing Office, 1978). "Task analysis" is the technique to teach the putting on of the T shirt.

were helping Morris learn how to order things in time, they carefully pointed out the sequence of events to him. First, the egg is
whole. Then it is broken. First, the point of the nail is touching the
wood. Then, after hammering, the nail is in the wood. They found
many "first . . . then" examples in everyday life to point out to
Morris. It is necessary to place events in time and place, especially
time, in order to learn to speak. Later it will be necessary to place
things in space in order to read. Morris can be helped by first
experiencing concrete real world events which are stubbornly irreversible.

An Aphasic Child

Janet is a three-and-a-half-year-old child who does not speak at all.
Her parents think she understands them but does not seem to form
words herself. The speech examiner sees that Janet has the communication skills of a year-old baby. In other aspects she is also
somewhat immature. Her gait is that of a child who has just
learned to walk. The examiner then asks the parents if Janet ever
suffered a blow to the head or had a high fever. The parents say
no, in fact Janet has never really been sick. She certainly never had
an accident which could have damaged her brain. Of course there
was the time she drank the gasoline. . . . The speech examiner
gulped and asked what had happened. Janet had drunk a small
amount of gasoline which was in a cup to be used as fuel for a
mower. Unfortunately Janet's mother in her panic had induced
vomiting to get the gas out of the little girl's system. That had
turned out to be the wrong thing to do. The gasoline is not so
harmful to the stomach as it is to the lungs and the gas had been
breathed into Janet's lungs twice. The child was sick for a week
with what amounted to pneumonia caused by the gasoline fumes.
Janet had had great trouble breathing at the time, gasping and
choking, and her skin had turned blue. Janet's mother did not
think this could have had anything to do with her child's failure to
speak. However, after further interviewing, the speech examiner
found out that Janet had been speaking in two-word sentences
until, when she was sixteen months, the awful gasoline incident
had happened. Most probably the child had suffered brain damage
during that period when she was having trouble breathing. The
brain needs oxygen more urgently than the rest of the body, and so

if there is a lack of air for any reason it is the brain that suffers first. Janet had suffered brain damage just as though she had had a blow to her head or a convulsion from a high fever.[10]

A person of any age can suffer brain damage due to an injury. Aphasia occurs when a person who has had language suffers brain damage and speech and language are impaired. The term "aphasia" is also used when people have strokes resulting in an inability to speak. Janet can be said to have aphasia, but since the damage was to a developing language system rather than to one already functioning, the problem Janet faces is quite like the problem faced by Nina or Morris. Since Janet is so young she can be trained to use the undamaged parts of her brain to learn language. She will need help. Although the cause is different, the problem and remedy are similar. Parents should remember that the most crucial speech organ in their children is the brain and that any damage to the brain can result in impaired speech. Lack of oxygen to the brain for any reason is cause for concern, especially in language functioning.

The Child Who Seems Brain-Injured

Andy is a handful. At four he is constantly on the go. He goes from one thing to another nonstop until he drops from exhaustion. It is more than his mother can do just to keep him from hurting himself and others. Now Andy is not just rambunctious or boisterous, normal characteristics for four-year-old boys, but seems driven by an inner frenzy. It is as if he cannot stop even if he wanted to. Andy's speech is not intelligible; he talks in sentences, but they are not coherent. He has problems in placing things in time and space, problems similar to Morris's.

Why was Andy so difficult to rear? Why wasn't he like other children? His parents were sure that their methods of upbringing were all wrong. They thought that if they could handle their son properly he could behave. They tried all sorts of child-rearing strategies. They tried being permissive, letting him act out and

10. Hubbell, op. cit. Even in Janet's case it seems obvious to point to the poisoning incident—but it is still merely a guess at the cause. When dealing with large groups of children, it can be shown that incidents such as Janet's are more frequent in the language-disabled children's histories than in the population as a whole, but whether such statistical evidence points to *the* cause is another matter.

express himself. They were not going to try to control his behavior in any way. This regimen proved to be impossible. He was a danger to himself and to others unless there were some constraints on his behavior. Then they tried being very strict. They would set definite limits and punish him severely and promptly when he acted up. They found that they spent most of the day punishing him and yet his behavior did not change. They tried a different diet, one with no sugar or soft drinks, and still there was no change in Andy's behavior. Baby sitters shunned the family so that the parents did not even get an occasional evening out. Not only was his behavior unruly and impossible to control, but they were worried that he was not learning as he should. Andy's parents noticed that their son did not speak as clearly as other children his age. Not only were his words not pronounced properly but he did not seem to know as many words as other children did. His sentences seemed fragmented. They were not sure that Andy could hear because he often did not answer when his name was called. The pediatrician suggested that Andy be seen by a neurologist.

Andy was given a complete neurological workup. All the tests came out negative; that is, there was no brain damage which could be found by direct examination. Nevertheless the doctor said that Andy seemed like a child who had undergone brain injury.

Minimal Brain Dysfunction (MBD)

Such a child, one whose brain damage is inferred from his behavior, is sometimes called minimally brain damaged or more accurately someone with minimal brain dysfunction (MBD). The reasons for MBD are not known, and there is some argument over them. Some say there is physical damage but so slight that the tests and measuring methods available are not subtle enough to detect it. Others think that it is a type of brain disability that we do not understand and so do not know how to search for, such as some chemical or enzyme imbalance in the brain. If we understood the chemistry of the brain and how it affects behavior, we would know what to look for. Some others think it is mainly a psychological problem brought on by certain emotional events. There is also a group who believe that MBD is the outcome of the modern American diet full of chemical additives and overly processed foods. But even the prevalence of MBD is difficult to pinpoint. Some authorities claim that 15 percent of schoolchildren show some signs of MBD while more conservative estimators put the percentage at 2 percent. The difference in these surveys must at least in part be due to the definition of MBD symptoms and how severe they must be to be counted. Many children are impulsive, have low attention spans, are fidgety, have speech problems, have perceptual problems, don't consider the consequences of their actions and are distractable. How severe one of these MBD signs has to be to be included remains an area of disagreement.

Still Andy's parents were relieved to know that their son's condition, whatever its origin, was not caused by their failure as parents. A great burden of guilt was lifted from them. They also learned that what had seemed to be two separate problems, the behavior and the speech, were in fact different aspects of the same condition. Andy was not able to learn well partly because of his extreme distractability. Many things that young children learn on their own take more than a half minute of attention. Most children do not concentrate on problems for hours on end, but a four-year-old child should be able to attend to something interesting for three to five minutes.

Helping the MBD Child

The neurologist suggested a special school for Andy where there would be experts in special education and language pathologists to help him with his speech. Andy's parents were delighted to find a preschool that would take him. They learned various valuable techniques for handling him effectively.

They found that Andy could concentrate on one thing better if there was only one thing in view. They learned to put all the other toys away and give him only one toy to play with at a time. They tried to keep his room as free from distractions as possible by putting other toys and objects out of view. They found that Andy was better able to play with one child at a time than with a group of children. Since Andy had trouble in figure-ground discrimination, the whole world was a distracting background concealing whatever he was supposed to pay attention to. His parents developed a very structured schedule for Andy. They gave up making spontaneous spur-of-the-moment decisions to do something. Whenever routine was to be broken, for a holiday or a relative's visit, it was planned and discussed in detail. The parents felt that their life style was somewhat cramped, but it did seem to help Andy. The neurologist prescribed some medication for Andy as a temporary aid to getting him to calm down to enter a remedial program at home and at school. Ironically the drug prescribed acts as a stimulant for most adults.

It is not completely understood why these drugs have such a seemingly contrary effect upon children like Andy. Perhaps it stimulates one's ability to organize activity and more organized behavior looks like calmer behavior to others. The drug seemed to increase Andy's ability to focus and pay attention, but the drug therapy was short term, and the dosage was gradually decreased to zero after two months. Andy's parents had to remain calm when Andy was bursting with activity. They had to respond to his disorganized behavior with their superorganized behavior. When Andy became overemotional, they had to be calm and dispassionate. They were careful to use simple sentences with Andy, as do the parents of other language delayed children.

Andy's parents found that once they had learned to control Andy's behavior or, more accurately, once they had developed Andy's ability to control his own behavior, his speaking and understanding increased. They discovered that their child could learn but not under circumstances brought about by his uncontrolled behavior. There are definitely other learning disabilities for Andy to overcome, but achieving control over his behavior is the first step.

An Autistic Child

Eva is a very strange child. She is beautiful and physically perfect, but at six years of age she does not really communicate with other people at all. Her occasional use of speech is more like the other activities she does by herself: banging her head against the wall or rocking in her rocking chair for hours on end. It seems a private communication, a message to herself alone. Eva's parents knew that she was different from the first few weeks of her life. Most babies (even babies who have severe handicaps like Nina, Karl, Morris or Andy) fit themselves into their parent's arms as they are held. When Eva's mother would pick her up when she was a few weeks old she would stiffen as if she were resisting being held and cuddled. Eva's mother felt that her baby did not like her. As time went on, Eva did not seem responsive to people around her. Her parents thought at first that she was deaf. A hearing examination at one year showed that her ears were fine. In fact Eva often listened to music and would hum the tune afterward. There were a few sound-making toys that Eva liked very much and played with a great deal. But still she made no attempt to talk nor did she appear to understand what other people said. It seemed to her parents that she had no desire to talk. Moreover, she did not seem to recognize her parents from other adults. Although she seemed uninterested in the people around her she seemed passionately interested in ritual and routine. Bedtime and mealtime had to follow the exact same procedure every day. If Eva's clothes were put into a different place she would fly into a screaming tantrum. At about two years of age Eva began to say a few words but only one at a time. At five years Eva could say a few more words but still never more than one at a time. Eva is an autistic child.

Controversy over the Cause of Autism

Autism is a widely misunderstood condition in children. It was first identified in the 1940s and thought to be an emotional disorder. It is an understandable conclusion to come to. Autistic children have a lack of affective or emotional behavior which is difficult to understand. It was assumed that autism resulted from parental rejection ("refrigerator mothers"), that affective behavior was learned and that if a child were rejected emotionally a child would never learn to relate to other people. The lack of language was seen as merely one outcome of this emotional disorder. Needless to say, the parents (especially mothers) of autistic children were made to feel pretty guilty. Because Eva rejected being picked up from the time she was a few weeks old, her mother did not cuddle her as much as she would have a normal baby. When the psychiatrist tried to probe the reasons she rejected her child, she thought that perhaps she *had* rejected the baby. In the past few years the thinking on autism has completely turned around. Eva's parents learned a great deal from the parents' group they joined. Autism is a severe language disorder, maybe the most severe. Children like Eva do not seem programmed as other children are to pair their life experience with a language code. This inborn language capacity is such a basic part of the human makeup that when we see a child who lacks it, the result is very strange and puzzling. An autistic person has a hard time functioning in the world.[11] By understanding what an autistic child experiences, we understand better how vital and important language is. Language makes our lives more interesting and richer but most importantly is vital to our survival.

Understanding the Autistic Child's Behavior

Eva's parents learned that the reason Eva insisted on ritual, rigidly doing the same thing the same way every day, was that the world was frighteningly confusing to her. The only hope she had of making any sense out of her surroundings was by having them so predictable that she knew them by rote. One small change, however, would throw her back into chaos. She would play with the same toy hours on end, deriving comfort in sameness. Eva's parents noticed that her words were very concrete, the names of tangible things and specific things. For instance, she used the word *shoe* to refer to her shoes, which were made of brown leather. She did not generalize the word to cover tennis shoes or sandals, nor did she seem to understand that the word *shoe* could be used for mother's high-heeled pumps or father's loafers. An autistic child does not seem to surround words with meanings, functions (what you use shoes for) or the class of thing they belong to (shoes are articles of clothing). All the word *shoe* could do was to stand for one particular shoe. Language cannot be so restricted. One day Eva's mother was driven to distraction by Eva's playing the same little tune on her toy xylophone for several hours and she exclaimed "Cut it out!" Eva then solemnly brought her a pair of scissors. This was not a joke—it was a very literal mind at work.

Helping an Autistic Child

Can autistic children be cured? As far as we know there is no cure for autism, but these children can be helped. Early attempts

11. L. Wing, *Autistic Children: A Guide for Parents and Professionals* (Secaucus, NJ: The Citadel Press, 1980). One estimate of the prevalence of autism is between four and five children out of ten thousand, as prevalent as profound deafness and more prevalent than total blindness.

to treat the emotional disorder were failures, not only because it is probably not an emotional disorder in the first place but because the method of psychological treatment is through talk. Talking to these children about feelings (which they do not understand because emotions are too abstract) only confuses them. And since confusion is painful to them, psychological treatment only increases their distress. Most autistic children are mentally retarded. Even those with areas of intellectual competence are impaired in their learning because of their limited language and are therefore functionally retarded.

By going back to the one-word level of language and slowly building from there it is possible to help autistic children communicate. Often the spoken words are combined with manual gestures which are easier for the child to grasp. The child can be led not only to words standing for concrete objects but can learn to group these words by function or color. With some ability in language, an autistic child will be able to clear up some of the confusion. As Eva progressed in her special education group, she became less rigid about her surroundings. She will probably never be able to understand the meaning of a saying like "A bird in the hand is worth two in the bush" as anything but a literal evaluation of the relative value of birds.

Not enough is understood about autism. Some theories about what causes it are based on biological difference in the brain but such a difference has not been found. We understand that these children are fearful, but we do not really know why. We observe that autistic children set different values on experiences than we do without our regard for consequences. For instance, some autistic children get pleasure out of breaking glass. They are not trying to be destructive, but the sound of the tinkling seems to mean something special. Eva and other children like her seem to live in a world of their own. They are an enigma to themselves and others.[12]

12. The mother of an autistic child speculated that the tales of "wolf children" or "wild children" supposedly brought up by wild animals and therefore without language were probably autistic children abandoned by their parents. It is not that the children did not talk because they were abandoned, but were abandoned because they were difficult to raise—part of the difficulty being lack of language. She also pointed out that the lead character of the movie *Being There*, played by the late Peter Sellers, was really an autistic adult who functioned at a high level. The movie is a fairly accurate portrayal of how an autistic person interacts with the world.

Helping Your Child Build a Language

In Chapter 1 you learned a normal child builds a language. You were given suggestions to help the process along. They are effective and fun to do; the parent of a normal child can enjoy taking an active part in the language learning. If your child is normal, however, it is not absolutely necessary for you to take *any* part in helping or teaching other than your usual everyday speech and conversation which serve as the raw material for your child's language. Many children have had parents who were not particularly concerned about their language development; but the children learned to talk. Nature did not make it necessary for parents to take an active effort to teach their children to talk; most pick it up on their own. But if your child is not talking spontaneously it is absolutely necessary that you actively help.

If you suspect that your child is not learning language normally, there are several things you should do. First take your child to a speech/language pathologist to determine whether or not there is a problem. If there is nothing wrong with your child, the time and money will have been well spent for the peace of mind it gives you. If the speech/language pathologist does find a problem, you and your child can and should get to work on it right away. If the speech/language pathologist does not give your child a hearing examination, you should take your child to an audiologist to see if there is enough hearing for language development. If your child does need therapy or remediation, take an active part in the program to give it the best chance of succeeding. If the remedial program is through the public schools, be sure to go to the scheduled conferences with the special education teachers. Visit the class often to keep up with what is going on in your child's therapy.

There are many different things you can do at home to help your child who is having difficulty learning language. To begin with, you can simplify your own speech. It may be necessary to limit your sentences to three or four words if you want your language-disabled child to understand everything you say. It would also be helpful if you could simplify some of the speech you have with other members of the family when your child is present. Children learn from listening to general conversation as well as from conversation directed at themselves. It would help your child to be able to make sense out of overheard conversation. Try to demonstrate what you are saying as you say it by using more gestures in your speech. Use your child's sense of touch when appropriate, letting the child squeeze a pillow while you explain it is soft. If your child has trouble processing a message coming in through the ears, help by using the eyes and fingers to receive it. If your child has trouble following a spoken message, it may take more time than usual to process it. Most of us assume that comprehension is simultaneous with the speech of the talker but your child may need more time to receive the message and figure out what it means. Sometimes the child will repeat the message in order to hold on to it long enough. It is often helpful if you repeat what you just said. You must remind yourself that you need to repeat, not because your child was not listening to you the first time but because listening is a very difficult task for your child and takes a little time. To help your child comprehend easier, follow through on your requests: if you ask your child to do something, make sure that it gets done. When you tell your child to eat a sandwich in the kitchen, see to it that the child does eat it in the kitchen and not in the living room. There is a tendency for parents to tell a child to do something and then either ignore or punish disobedience. But if your child is language-disordered, you want to clarify both the meaning of your request and teach the child attentiveness. Making sure your child does exactly what you say is the way to be sure that the child comprehended it.

Whether or not your child is receiving professional help, some language development is going on even though it seems slower than for normal boys and girls. As your child learns, several stages of behavior are going on at once. You will hear the new and more mature attempt at language one minute, and the next minute there will be a reversion to the old baby ways such as pointing and grunting instead of asking for the object by name. By responding only to the mature types of communication and being unresponsive to the immature styles, your child will be encouraged to use the mature means of communication. Don't punish or scold your child for using baby methods; just see to it that they don't work. It is worth the patience it takes to give your child a chance to say "I want the ball" rather than pointing to it. Don't expect the most advanced part of your child's repertoire of behavior when the child is tired or sick.

If your child is learning disabled as part of the language problem, you may find that altering the environment is helpful. Your child will be able to do a task better if there are as few distractions as possible. When your child wants to color, set up the table with only the crayons and paper, clearing off all the other things that are not needed. Limit the number of crayons as well. Encouraging your child to conduct a mature conversation will be easier without other people and without the distraction of the television or the radio. In these quiet times you can ask the child to talk to you about the latest art creations or block buildings. When your child wants to talk to you be sure to listen closely. It is discouraging for a child who is having problems organizing words into speech to feel that the parent's attention is wandering.

When you are trying to get your child to express thoughts in words, encourage open-ended discussion. Avoid yes and no questions. If you look at your child's picture and ask, "Is that a boat?" the child will answer yes or no and nothing else. If you say, "Tell me about your picture," your child will have to be creative with words as well as with a paintbrush. If you must ask questions to keep the conversation going, ask questions that begin with who, what, why, where, when, how—questions that cannot be answered with just a yes or no.

As recently as a generation ago, educators did not recognize that it was possible to have a specific developmental language disorder. Aphasias were recognized long before, but until modern medicine, most people who suffered head wounds severe enough to affect language did not live long enough to have a communication problem. The children who had developmental disorders of language for any reason were simply considered mentally retarded (classified as feeble-minded or idiots, imbeciles or morons) and thought uneducable. The workings of the thinking process were not well enough understood to separate various types of development. There is still much we do not understand about the workings of the mind, and perhaps we will never understand them completely. We are finding that there are many lines of intellectual development. Even the term "language development" is too broad. Many processes are involved in a functioning language: perceptual skills, short-term memory, long-term memory, motor skills (ability to form speech), social skills, psychological development, ability to control behavior. All these factors have to be put together, and so we must include integrative skills. Many of these processes are learned, although in the main, they do not need to be taught. As we become aware of the complexity of language, a concept so familiar that it is usually overlooked by people as too ordinary to be interesting, we are able to discover the precise areas of trouble that an individual child may have and then teach the particular skill to the child.

Language disorders in children also provide researchers with a laboratory situation. They can then answer questions such as how a deficiency in visual perception affects a child's vocabulary. These questions are asked to understand how normal children learn to talk as well as how communicatively handicapped children can be helped. Perhaps some of these disorders might turn out to be preventable. The outlook for the language-disordered child is far better than it was in the past and even more optimistic in the future.

Suggestions for the Parents of Language-Delayed Children

- Don't demand perfect pronunciation.
- Encourage your child to speak even if it doesn't come out right.
- Expand your child's incomplete attempt to say something to give the child a model of what the complete utterance is.
- Keep your own sentences simple and short.
- Repeat yourself to give your child a chance to understand.
- Try to avoid figures of speech which might be confusing such as "a bolt from the blue" or "raining cats and dogs."
- Give your child a chance to say what is wanted before giving it— don't be too understanding.
- Encourage your child to imitate your speech without insisting on it.
- Combine your words with gestures to aid understanding.
- Try to keep your child's play area free of distraction; encourage play with one toy at a time.
- Talk about what you are doing.
- Talk about what your child is doing.
- Take your child places. Discuss them before, during and after the outings.
- Emphasize the proper order of things: "First put on your socks and then put on your shoes."

- Try to simplify your child's sensory input. For instance, turn off television while carrying on a conversation.
- Mean what you say to aid the child's understanding. If you say you will do something, do it.
- Be consistent in your discipline.
- Get professional help for your child.
- Observe clinic sessions if possible.
- Continue clinic activities at home with clinician's advice.

4

Can Your Child Hear?

Why Doesn't Your Child Talk?

The relationship between deafness and speaking has not always been understood. In the Middle Ages and even into modern times, those who were dumb (a term originally meaning mute) were thought to be unable to talk because somehow their speech was blocked. It was assumed they could hear. The term "dumb" came to be a synonym for stupid because these speechless persons did not react intelligently to questions from others. The connection between speech and hearing was not clear.

Jeremy has just celebrated his second birthday. A handsome, lively child, sometimes a little hard to control, he seems very bright. But why doesn't he talk? Most children his age say at least a few words; some say considerably more. Jeremy doesn't even try to say *Mama* or *Dada*. He makes vowel-like noises, but they are not at all like speech. But he doesn't seem dull or stupid—he just doesn't talk. Jeremy's mother has been worried about his hearing. He does not seem to respond to his name, and he won't or cannot respond to the simplest requests. Yet, she had been assured at the last medical check-up that there was nothing to worry about. The doctor had clapped loudly behind Jeremy's back and the child had obviously reacted with a startled jump. Jeremy's parents, however, were not completely satisfied. They took him to be tested at a speech and hearing clinic even though his doctor had said that he was too young for such a test. They found that Jeremy had a moderate to severe hearing loss. He could hear certain loud noises such as a door slamming and possibly a shout if the shouter were right next to him. (This was how he was able to hear the clap behind his back.) In short, although able to hear some sound, Jeremy was cut off from the sound of other people's voices. Jeremy didn't talk because he had never heard anyone else talk. Hearing loss does not have to be complete to impair a child's language learning. Jeremy may have been able to hear a few speech sounds or parts of words when they were spoken loudly very near him. But this would not be enough to teach him how to talk.

Jeremy's parents took him to a doctor specializing in diseases of the ear. They hoped that an operation might restore his hearing but were disappointed to learn that there was no operation to help Jeremy. His hearing loss was permanent. Then they investigated hearing aids. Jeremy's grandmother had recently gotten a hearing aid for the type of hearing loss that often comes with age. They reasoned that just as some children have to wear glasses to see properly, Jeremy would have to wear a hearing aid to hear properly. The parents were disappointed again. Hearing aids, unlike glasses, cannot without difficulty be made to compensate precisely for the sounds that are not heard. A hearing aid is a help but not a cure. Jeremy's grandmother had already learned to talk and could be trained to use the aid to help her understand, although she was the first to admit that hearing through a hearing aid was not like the real thing. The problem of maintaining communication after losing hearing when you have already learned to talk is quite different from having to build your own language on the distorted and muffled speech you could hear through the aid. Jeremy's parents were told that he was too young to be fitted with a hearing aid or to wear one. He could not be tested accurately enough to get a proper selection and would not be able to take care of any aid with which he was fitted. His parents were told to wait until Jeremy was older before trying a hearing aid.

Hearing Loss at an Early Age

Early Testing for a High-Risk Baby

Brenda is eight months old. Brenda's mother had a mild infection during her pregnancy which might have been German measles (or rubella). She thought that her baby might have a hearing problem as well as eye and heart problems. When Brenda was born she was examined carefully and found to be free of the eye and heart disorders which are often consequences of maternal rubella. Brenda gooed and gurgled at three months, just as normal babies do; nevertheless Brenda's pediatrician wanted her to have a hearing examination. At the speech and hearing clinic, Brenda's parents found that, as best as could be determined at this age, their baby had a very severe hearing loss. The parents took her home in silence. Brenda's mother bathed her without the usual accompanying song. Brenda's father stopped talking to her. When the other members of the family learned about Brenda's handicap they also stopped talking or singing to her. Luckily the week following the hearing test they had an appointment with the audiologist (a specialist in the treatment of hearing disorders) in order to plan Brenda's early education. The audiologist told Brenda's family to stop the silent treatment; if anything Brenda needs *more* not less sound. The audiologist explained that Brenda could learn to talk normally and to listen with amplification if the parents were willing to work very hard with her and to get to work on it immediately. In addition to all the care that Brenda's parents normally would give her they would have to give her the sound that she couldn't pick up naturally. They would be helped by electronics. Even a child with a hearing loss like Brenda's has enough hearing to experience some sound. Brenda was then fitted with a special hearing aid. This was not the tiny invisible aid often worn by older people. It was a little vest made of canvas which contained the working parts of the aid.

Wires went to both ears. The aid was somewhat of a contraption, but Brenda soon took it in stride. Brenda and her parents signed up for a home demonstration program. The "clinic" looked like a regular house where clinicians, mothers, fathers and some grandparents all worked together bringing the sounds of normal life to their hearing-impaired children. Because the sounds Brenda heard were less perfect than those heard by a fully hearing child, Brenda's parents had to create more sound stimulation. Fortunately they started early enough so that Brenda will be able to learn her language at the normal language learning age. Brenda will receive auditory training in which the clinician or her parents will direct her attention to certain sounds in the environment. As she gets older they will engage in listening and imitating games. Later there will be emphasis on speech sounds hard to hear even with amplification. There will be activities designed to give Brenda a greater than normal exposure to these sounds and words.

Monitoring and Caring for the Hearing Aid

The hearing specialist told Brenda's parents that the hearing aids were not as good as they would like them to be because it is so difficult to test hearing accurately at Brenda's age (very much what Jeremy's parents were told). Nevertheless even this imperfect sound will enable Brenda to develop her language naturally. Her parents observed her more carefully than parents of normal children to note any changes in her behavior in order to judge how well her hearing aid was working. After putting the hearing aid on Brenda, her mother or father spoke to her in a normal tone of voice. If she blinked her eyes or showed signs of discomfort, the parent knew that the volume was too high. If the baby did not turn toward the speaking parent, the volume was too soft. They were told that it was very important to keep the hearing aid at the right volume for Brenda all the time. In addition they had to be sure to keep plenty of spare batteries (like electronic wristwatch batteries) on hand because they have a short lifetime. The parents had to keep the ear molds (the buttons that fit into the ear) clean and fitting properly as Brenda grew.

Although Jeremy has somewhat more hearing ability than Brenda, the outlook for Brenda's learning to talk like everyone else is brighter than his. Jeremy has missed a great deal of his language learning time and is still missing his needed sound stimulation with each day of delay. He can start in now with amplification, but those early months of becoming acquainted with the sensation of hearing are lost forever along with the fantastic learning rate of a young infant.

Hearing: The Underestimated Sense

The Handicap of Hearing Loss

Both Jeremy and Brenda have sensorineural hearing losses, sometimes called nerve deafness. They were born with the problem, and there is no medical cure. The estimates are that three to six babies out of one thousand live births have inborn hearing loss. A considerably greater number of children (one million) in the United States have some degree of hearing handicap. There are several types of hearing loss, depending on what part of the ear is damaged. Some types of hearing loss can be helped by medical treatment and/or surgery, but others cannot be changed.

Many of us don't always recognize how much a handicap deafness can be. We tend to be more fearful of blindness than hearing loss. Being unable to see certainly would be devastating, but unlike deafness it does not cut you off from human contact. The isolation caused by deafness is even more difficult to adjust to. We are vision-oriented, perhaps because we see modern life being more dependent on vision than hearing, and we take our hearing for granted. Under more primitive conditions we might have found our hearing to be more useful for getting around as well as for communication. Before reading became widespread, we were educated more through our ears than our eyes. It was the church bell that told us when to quit work, not a watch. A hunter in the forest depends more on his ears to detect game than his eyes.

Not only do we often underestimate how useful hearing is, we are often unaware of how remarkable are its workings. We can hear a great range of sounds from very high pitched to low. With some exceptions the smaller the animal the higher the pitch to which it is sensitive. My cat can hear a much higher-pitched sound than I can, and I can hear a much higher-pitched sound than an elephant can. The range of soft to loud sounds our ears can hear is amazingly wide. If you converted sound energy into light energy, and if your eyes were as good as your ears, you could see a thirty-watt light bulb in Chicago from Nashville (if you could get a clear view).[1] And this is just everyday sensitivity. You can also tolerate sounds one hundred billion times as powerful as the softest sounds you can hear.

The Outer and Middle Ear

Your ear is an incredibly complex organ. The part of the ear you see is not the part of the ear you hear with. The main function of the outer ear is to protect the working part of the ear. A canal leads from the outer ear to the eardrum. The eardrum divides the outer ear from the middle ear. Sound waves are a series of pressure waves that move from a sound source like ripples on water when you drop a stone into a pond. These air pressure waves hit the thin-membrane eardrum, which moves every time a pressure wave hits it. The faster the waves come the higher pitched the sound. The stronger the pressure waves the louder the sound. On the other side of the eardrum are the little bones of the ear. They are the smallest bones in the body, each as small as a grain of rice. The middle ear which houses this series of bones is a tiny chamber filled with air. (When your ear hurts in an airplane, it is because the pressure in the middle ear cannot change as quickly as the air pressure on the outside. We can bear barometric changes in the weather but not air travel.) A tube connects this part of the ear with the throat and nasal cavity in order to equalize the pressure in and out of the middle ear. When you get a cold or hay fever, the middle ear gets congested the same way your nose gets stopped up and you don't hear as well as usual. Your middle ear, nose and throat are all connected. Small children with short heads are therefore most likely to get ear congestion from postnasal drip and are more susceptible to ear infections, earaches and hearing loss from middle ear problems. If the ear trouble is in the middle ear there are many medical procedures available, not only to relieve hearing loss but to prevent it.

1. This calculation was done by my husband, John Barach, a professor of physics. My colleagues were as intrigued by it as I was. Of course you would need a clear view free of other lights to see the thirty-watt bulb (if your eyes were as sensitive as your ears). You can hear a pin drop only in a quiet room.

The Inner Ear—Where Hearing Takes Place

Important as it is, the middle ear is not the real organ of hearing. The sound pressure waves pass through this tiny chamber to be transferred by an intricate hydraulic and lever system to an even smaller chamber, the inner ear. Even if the middle ear were completely eliminated or damaged and the inner ear still intact there would be some hearing. In such a case the person would have lost the conduction or transference to the inner ear and would suffer what is called a conductive hearing loss. The inner ear houses both the hearing organ and the mechanism by which you can keep your balance and know which way is up and which way is down. The whole inner ear chamber is filled with liquid and sealed off from the middle ear. Therefore the real function of the middle ear is to transfer the sound from air to liquid. The only communication between the middle and the inner ear is an oval window. One of the tiny bones presses against the membrane covering this window each time a sound wave passes through. The sound receptors are a series of little hairlike cells inside a snailshell-shaped tube. When the liquid inside the inner ear is rippled from pressure on the oval window, the little hairs move and this in turn sends electrical signals through the auditory nerve to the brain. You spend the first few months and years of your life learning to interpret these signals as noise, music, talk. If the damage to the ear is in either this inner ear or the nerve which goes from the hearing organ to the brain, the loss is known as a sensorineural hearing loss. Sometimes a person can have damage in both the middle and the inner ear, in which case the person has a mixed loss. An audiologist can determine what kind of loss there is.[2] In general a sensorineural loss is beyond the ability of surgery or medicine to cure. If your child has been diagnosed as having a

2. An audiologist can tell the difference between a sensorineural hearing loss and a conductive loss because there are two sound stimulus points, one at the opening of the ear canal and the other directly on the bone behind the ear. If a patient responds to direct bone stimulation (bypassing the middle ear) and not to the air (sound into the ear canal), there is a conductive loss. If the patient responds to neither bone nor air there is sensorineural loss. If the patient needs a louder than normal sound to respond to bone stimulation but an even louder sound to respond to air stimulation, there is a mixed loss, that is, both middle and inner ear are impaired. If the patient's responses are reduced for bone stimulation but more reduced for air, there is a mixed loss that is both middle and inner ear are impaired.

sensorineural hearing loss, the treatment for your child is to learn to live with it and communicate in spite of it.

Medical Advances and Hearing Loss

In the days before antibiotics a great many people had conductive hearing losses left over from childhood infections. They still exist in our middle-aged population. Many had lost their hearing after they had learned to talk and although they have been inconvenienced by impaired hearing all their lives, the learning of and understanding of their own language have not been damaged. People with this type of hearing loss are pretty good candidates for the amplification hearing aids can provide. There were a number of surgical procedures which were used not only to cure conductive hearing losses but to save the patient from possible spread of infection to the brain. With antibiotics there is no reason for an ear infection to develop to such a drastic state. Other conditions of the middle ear can be corrected surgically, especially with some of the new techniques of microsurgery.

Today, however, there are more sensorineural deaf and hard of hearing than before. Many of these youngsters who might not have lived even a decade ago were saved at birth because of modern medical advances. Hearing loss is more common among children who were born prematurely than those who were born at full term. Medical procedures have saved more children from life-threatening illnesses than ever before, but the disease can leave a hearing loss in its wake. Sometimes the treatment itself creates a hearing impairment as an aftereffect. The irony is that modern medicine has left us with a greater number of untreatable hearing losses.

The Connection Between Hearing Loss and Speech

It is very difficult to identify hearing loss in a baby or a young child. A parent has to infer indirectly from the child's behavior and often just has to guess whether or not the child is hearing properly. A person who has been able to hear will miss it if it is lost. But a child who has never heard doesn't know what sound is and won't miss what was never experienced. Such a child cannot talk and tell you why moving your lips and mouth around doesn't make any sense. Years can pass without your realizing that your child cannot hear.

What the Hard-of-Hearing Child Can and Cannot Hear

Jeremy's father is still puzzled. If the baby couldn't hear, why did he jump when the doctor clapped loudly behind his back? Both parents feel that Jeremy responded to rhythm in music when they played their stereo. The answer is the kind of hearing loss Jeremy has. Hearing losses are measured by how severe they are; that is, how loud a sound has to be before the person can hear it at all. With Jeremy's loss he would just about be able to hear the noise of a school cafeteria but not the background noise of a carpeted and elegant restaurant. Hearing losses are also measured by which type of sounds are heard. With Jeremy's type of impairment the high sounds are more difficult to hear than the lower-pitched sounds. The high notes on the piano would be harder for Jeremy to hear than the low notes, if any of them would be loud enough for him to hear at all. Thus if you amplify the sound signal for the child, giving each type of sound an equal gain, the low notes will come in too loud if the high notes can be heard at all. This will distort speech, and it will not sound to Jeremy anything like it sounds to normal-hearing people. "Three fishes in the pond" may sound like "Ree i'uh in uh on'." The vowels come through, but many of the consonants are omitted. Anyone would have a hard time learning to talk if that were the way speech sounded.[3] An audiologist can test hearing at various frequencies (pitches) and measure the degree of loss at each pitch. It is possible to fit a hearing aid to compensate for the frequencies that are impaired, but the state of the art is by no means perfect. It is not at all like glasses which can be ground to compensate for the individual features of the eyeball. Although some sound can be delivered to Jeremy through amplification, electronics will not provide him with normal hearing. If perfect compensation were possible, a deaf or hard-of-hearing child would be able to experience normal hearing and if fitted with an aid early enough could develop speech

---

3. Most sounds we hear are made of many tones (notes), some high and some low. Environmental sounds would also be distorted if there were reduced sensitivity in part of the sound spectrum. Since environmental sounds are mostly alerting mechanisms, that is significant by presence or absence not accuracy, such distortion is not so handicapping.

normally. At the present state of the art Jeremy could hear distorted speech. But it is a poor speech model to learn from unless given special help to overcome the disadvantages of such a model.

Hearing Loss That Grows Worse with Time

A high-risk baby, thirteen-month-old Mario falls into a group of hearing-handicapped children about whom there is a great deal of controversy over treatment. Mario's parents were very concerned with his hearing because Mario's mother had a brother who had been deaf from birth. With such an inheritance Mario's parents realized that he was a high-risk baby and they had his hearing screened with a new hearing screening technique at the hospital when he was a month old. He passed the test with flying colors. The parents breathed a sigh of relief, feeling secure that their child's hearing was normal. Mario cooed and gurgled and made all the delightful little noises that his two older sisters had made. At five months Mario was interested in a rattle his grandmother had brought him, but not when the rattle was shaken out of his sight. Mario's mother did not worry because she had observed that he always turned toward her when she spoke to him. As the months went on, however, Mario's cooing and gurgling did not change. He might go "kuh" but he never went "kuh kuh kuh" the way babies do in the second half of their first year. He was able to pull himself to a standing position at nine months and was quite good at taking things apart. At eleven months he could open every drawer in the house and take out all its contents. He needed discipline, but verbal disapproval, which had worked with the other children, seemed to have no effect. Physical intervention was the only way to stop Mario from continuing undesirable behavior. Mario never repeated sounds he heard. There wasn't even a hint of an attempted word. Worse, Mario did not respond to his own name. Mario's father remembered that the girls had understood their own names long before they had said anything.

Finally at the regular medical checkup they asked the doctor about Mario's disturbing behavior. After the examination the doctor recommended to Mario's parents that his hearing be tested again. They protested, feeling the question of Mario's hearing had been cleared up months ago. The doctor explained gently that sometimes a baby will have a progressive hearing loss, that Mario could have been born with normal hearing or enough hearing to pass the infant screening but that he could have had an inborn condition in which hearing is gradually lost. Sometimes the progressive hearing loss gives the child time to learn speech, but sometimes the loss proceeds more rapidly. Mario had responded to noises and sounds in the early months, but he was not responding to them now. Mario was taken to an audiologist the next week. The doctor's fears had turned out to be true. Mario had a profound hearing loss, less hearing than Brenda had. There was very little sound getting through his ears. If he were near enough he could hear a loud truck, a chain saw, a power saw, a jet plane taking off, a loud rock band or a large power mower. He would not be able to hear any speech sounds, radio or television. Mario's parents were told that there was no medical treatment to increase the child's hearing and that they would have to start education and therapy to teach him to live with his handicap. Communication would not come naturally to Mario; he would have to be taught some system which would enable him to express himself and learn and think about the world. Mario's parents had to decide upon which method to follow. In order to make this important decision Mario's parents had to examine their own feelings and beliefs about deafness.

Some Myths about Deafness That You May Believe

Just because we no longer think that deaf people are stupid does not mean that the term "deaf" still doesn't carry some harmful baggage.[4] Because these myths affect our way of treating the child labeled "deaf," often resulting in a distortion of that child's learning environment, let us examine these myths. This distortion in itself creates the outcome which reinforces the myth.

"There is little point in speaking to a deaf child." Any child treated with silence will be auditorily deprived and not learn to speak properly. The main reason for a deaf child to fail to learn to talk is auditory deprivation. If your child has residual hearing (more than three fourths of hearing-impaired children do), you

4. C. C. Weir, "Habilitation and Rehabilitation of the Hearing Impaired," from *Introduction to Communication Disorders*, ed. by T. J. Hixon, L. D. Shriberg and J. H. Saxman (Englewood Cliffs, NJ: Prentice-Hall, 1980). The "myths" of hearing impairment are an expansion of a list of assumed characteristics that go with the label of "deaf."

have taken that residual hearing away by your silent treatment. If your child has a hearing problem or if you just *suspect* that your child has a hearing problem, keep talking.

"All deaf children need a different type of communication." We have become more aware of manual language of the deaf. Some television programs employ a person using sign language interpreting the spoken message. I am glad that this means of communication is becoming more acceptable for those who need it. But for the majority of hearing-impaired children it is not necessary and it has many disadvantages. If your child has a moderate hearing loss don't jump to the conclusion that sign language is the *only* way your child can communicate.

"Your deaf child will need a special school, probably one away from home in another city." Most states have residential schools for the deaf. It is true that if a deaf or even hard-of-hearing child is not given the extra help to learn to communicate by the age of six, that child will present an educational problem. The public school has traditionally not met educational needs before the age of six. If a child with impaired hearing were kept home without any special care and no means for amplification, regular school would be impossible. Historically states have run only one school for the deaf children of that state, and so many of the children had to leave home to get any kind of education. How sad it must have been in the past for children to be taken to a strange place and left there by their parents. It is particularly poignant because there was probably no way for the parents to warn or prepare the child beforehand, not having the ability to communicate. Nowadays there are many school settings available to children with hearing handicaps, depending upon the individual's communication skills: residential schools, day schools for the hearing impaired, special classes within the regular school and mainstreaming (integration into normal classes). Often children work step by step through these various arrangements, entering finally into regular classes. New laws for the handicapped provide education for the hearing impaired in most states of the United States from the age of three. There is more information on these laws in Chapter 9.

"There is no use fitting a child with a hearing aid." Sometimes the parents of a hearing-handicapped child will be told to wait until the child is old enough to be tested properly and can wear a hearing aid. Jeremy's parents were discouraged from fitting him with a hearing aid. It is true that your six-month-old baby

is hard to test for hearing. Not even you, the parent, can be sure what your baby's responses mean. Is the baby blinking in response to the noise you just made? Or just blinking? How can anybody possibly fit a hearing aid on such a little baby? (Even the hearing loss cannot be accurately measured.) Most physicians and audiologists find working with babies very difficult and are all too willing to postpone hearing assessment until an easier age to work with. Moreover, specialists realize that even under the best testing conditions, and with the most advanced hearing aids, the sound is not perfect. Still, some sound is better than none. Some talk getting through is better than none. Parents can learn to read their child's responses to sound and adjust the hearing aid guided by how the child behaves. As a parent you might be put off by the strange-looking machinery and not wish to attach it to your baby. The little vests holding the aids may seem bizarre at first sight, but your baby will get used to it faster than you. Some experts believe that it is better to get started with hearing aids on a baby before the child notices too much of the surroundings. Babies who have worn aids from four to six months of age probably accept them as a natural part of their bodies.

"Deaf persons will not succeed academically or be able to get good jobs." There is no reason that deaf people cannot succeed academically or at work. Of course either of these accomplishments requires some adjustment and working around the handicap. The myth persists because many children have been as handicapped by the preceding first four myths as by their deafness. Regular school becomes more difficult for your child not only because of poor hearing but because the lack of the spoken language makes reading almost impossible to learn. With all these obstacles lack of academic and vocational achievement would hardly be surprising. If, however, you discover the hearing loss early, and you intervene as soon as possible, fitting your child with hearing aids before the speech learning time, your child can succeed academically. People have been successful even without early intervention, but the odds are against it.

Seeking Help

Brenda and Jeremy fall into the two-thirds to three-fourths of hearing-handicapped children who have enough residual hearing so that normal speech and amplified hearing are not only possible but most desirable. Brenda is well on her way to living a normal life. As an adult she will probably take her place in society and her hearing loss will be known only because family and friends can see her hearing aid. Jeremy might never have completely normal speech. The longer his parents delay treating him the worse his speech will be. He is apt to speak in a monotone, or his speech may sound labored and heavy like a record played at too slow a speed. He might learn speech reading (the preferred term for lip reading because you look at the teeth, jaw, and tongue as well as the lips) and understand some regular speech. Only 20 to 30 percent of speech can be understood by speech reading alone so most successful speech readers combine speech reading with use of sound. He may use a combination of sign language and speech reading. Whatever Jeremy's ultimate method of communication will be, he will be more handicapped than necessary by the delay in treatment, a condition he will have to live with for the rest of his life. Remediation for Jeremy will include compensation for both lost language learning time as well as sensory impairment.

Oral-Auditory and Manual Language Approaches

Brenda and Jeremy have sensorineural hearing loss. Brenda's is more severe than Jeremy's, but like Jeremy's it is uneven; that is, worse in some frequencies than others. Why are Brenda's parents putting a hearing aid on her while knowing it is not a perfect compensation, and at an age when they wouldn't expect her to talk and understand even with normal hearing? If Jeremy's parents were discouraged from fitting him with an aid, why do Brenda's parents think it will help?

The difference in treatment and advice received by Brenda's parents and Jeremy's illustrates the opposing view in the education of hearing-impaired children. If you have a child with a hearing loss you must decide how to educate and handle the handicap. You can either become involved with a strictly oral-auditory program (speaking and hearing) or encourage your child to learn a manual language. The specialists are bitterly divided between the two approaches, and the controversy has been going on for years. There does not seem to be room for compromise, and so hearing-handicapped children and their parents are caught in the cross-fire of a professional dispute.

Treatment Methods

The various methods of treatment of the deaf are not different means to the same ends; the ends themselves are different. Mario's parents must choose not only *how* he will communicate with others, but with *whom* he will communicate. Basically there are two choices for Mario and his parents, although there are some modifications possible within each of these choices. One way to go would be to give up regular communication altogether and educate Mario totally in gesture language, using one of the manual systems available. The other choice is to give Mario some experience of sound through amplification and teach him to talk. If the residual sound is inadequate even with hearing aids to understand normal speech, Mario can learn speech reading. Mario's parents wanted to make the right decision, so they investigated both possibilities and even a third method called Total Communication which seemed a combination of both methods. Each specialist they visited claimed there was only one proper method to manage Mario's education— the method practiced by that particular specialist.

The argument in favor of sign language. They first visited a manualist. This sign and gesture proponent told Mario's parents that education of the deaf in this country has not been a success because there has been an insistence upon oral speech and auditory understanding. These are the impaired channels of communication. Mario is talented at many things—not only can he empty drawers, he is also a master at stacking plastic doughnuts on a spindle. Such manual coordination should serve him well in learning to sign. He seems more than usually observant of things that he sees, noticing small imperfections in objects that the rest of us would overlook. Careful observation is also necessary in comprehending sign language. He has spontaneously made up a few gestures of his own. Obviously signs and gestures are things he will be able to do. While it is true that the use of sign language will limit Mario to talking only with people who know sign language, at least he will be able to talk to someone. If the oral-auditory method is tried and fails, Mario will have nobody to talk to; he won't even have a language for thinking. Moreover, if Mario learns signing early he will be more skilled in it than if he waits until after he has tried and failed at oral-auditory communication. American Sign

Language, which is more related to spoken French than spoken English, is used worldwide, almost exclusively among deaf people and persons who work with the deaf. There are other types of sign language, some of which relate to English and are capable of using the same number of words as English is. The manualist went on to say that forcing Mario to use the type of communication he is least capable of would set him behind his contemporaries. He would never talk as well or understand as well as normal hearing people. But there is a whole communication system available in which Mario will not be handicapped. The greater current acceptance of handicapped people will not make it necessary for Mario to hide in a special deaf society as in time past. Mario's parents found these to be compelling arguments, but to explore the problem completely they kept the appointment they had made with the oral-auditory specialist.

The argument in favor of speech in spite of the difficulties. The oralist or verbalist countered every one of the manualist's arguments, pointing out that Mario had some residual hearing and that he could be given some sound stimulation through hearing aids. The totally deaf ear was rare. He would need to develop speech reading skills which would supplement his amplified hearing, but he was young enough to learn speech naturally. Normal speech and understanding through hearing and speech reading was a method which would not limit Mario to talking with only a few people. It is the natural language system which all human beings were designed to acquire. Language learning is intimately connected with intellectual development. The development of Mario's thinking processes would be enhanced by natural language learning. Manual language, moreover, would alienate Mario not only from his family, neighbors and culture but from most other Americans.

This is not to disparage American Sign Language or any of the other manual language systems. But it is true that a person growing up in the United States with a language different from English as his only language—be it Portuguese, Greek, Chinese or American Sign Language—is at a disadvantage. Furthermore even if manual language served Mario's needs to make contact with other people who conversed in that way, he would be handicapped in learning to read. Reading is based on the spoken language and would be very difficult for someone unfamiliar with the language beforehand. In manual language, gesture or sign is often the whole concept. Natural language includes rules of grammar as well as particular words. The verbalists claim that sign language does not really have a developed grammar. The sign language proponents take vigorous exception to this. Linguists (scientists who study the nature of language) debate the amount of grammar in sign language.[5] Nevertheless even if American Sign Language is as much a natural language as English, German or Japanese, it is a different language. The letters on the page confronting Mario when he started to learn to read would not have any relationship to the sign images he would have. The letters stand for the sound images that hearing people have in their minds; they then can translate the words they see to the speech they can hear (at least in their heads). Mario as a signer would be behind in reading and writing skills, two forms of communication which should be available to him. The verbalist explained that the writing done by students raised on sign language is usually below grade level. The compositions of high school students in residential schools for the deaf (where sign language is the method of communication) often show bizarre grammar although the spelling and penmanship is often very good. It is as if these children are writing in a different language from their own. If Mario learns English he will have only one system, one grammar to master, as well as being able to talk to anybody. Because of the degree of Mario's hearing disability, there is the possibility of cued speech to help his speech reading. It is difficult always to tell words apart by just seeing the speaker; for instance, *girl, curl* and *hurl* would be difficult to differentiate, but there are systems of cued speech that add gestures to help clear up such ambiguities.

The best of both systems? Total Communication. The verbalist's argument was pretty convincing. Mario's parents found themselves in a dilemma once more. They then heard about Total Communication, which promised the best of both worlds. Total

5. Sign language seems to spark controversy. In experiments investigating symbolic communication abilities of higher primates a modification of sign language was taught to chimpanzees. (Earlier attempts at teaching oral language to chimps had failed.) The chimps took to it—signed to their keepers and to each other. Conservatives scoffed at it, feeling that if chimpanzees do it it can't really be language. Some say that chimps are capable of language through appropriate channels, while others say it is not strictly symbolic language with a complete grammar. Probably people who use signs for communication have an internal grammar, but how clearly it can be expressed remains a point of controversy.

Communication is a term for various programs that use a combination of sign language, finger spelling (gestures which stand for each letter of an English word), speech, hearing aids and speech reading. Its attraction is that it is a means of opening up all channels of communication so that the child will be able to use the type that serves the particular needs of the moment. Many people are enthusiastic about this new technique. It is used in many school programs for the hearing impaired. It would be valuable for the child whose hearing handicap was discovered too late to help normal language learning. The easiest communication in such a case would be a manual system, which could be used to teach the child how to speak. But with a total communication program, the child would not be so cut off from the hearing population. Some people say that it may be like learning two primary languages at once, as when a child's parents live in a foreign country and the child picks up both the language of home and the language of the country. There is some controversy whether true bilingualism is an advantage or whether one or both of the languages suffer. Many professionals question TC. Rather than being a total solution for the hearing handicapped it may be more confusing and the level of communication lower than either the manual or the verbal. It may be hard to learn two languages at once and with TC the child might actually be learning several. It might be even more confusing if these languages were learned with different senses. Some TC programs stress more oral language than gesture, others put more stress on manual. Some oralists fear that the methods that were more difficult for the child to master would be quickly discarded in favor of the easier. Thus the notion of all channels being available for communication would not really hold true. Since the method is new there is no information on the long-term follow-up. The success or failure of the system will be known when there are many graduates of the program.[6]

6. Use of Total Communication is growing in American schools. Many are very enthusiastic. Probably the TC program does not produce the excellent expressive speech of many deaf persons trained verbally from a few months of age. I am not convinced that learning through different channels would be contradictory. With some mentally retarded people the gesture seems to reinforce rather than replace the spoken word (see Chapter 3).

Which Approach Is Best

Mario's parents finally decided to go with the approach that combined residual hearing and amplification-speech reading. They felt that Mario would have a better chance at a normal life if they could help him learn his language and theirs, realizing that they would have the primary teaching and therapy responsibilities in the early and most important years. Since neither parent had any experience in the treatment of the handicapped, they needed special training. One or both parents would take Mario to the clinic three times a week, working with him as the clinician watched. The clinician would then discuss the session with the parent. Sessions were devoted to helping the parents learn to care for the hearing aid. Not only did Mario's parents have to learn to take care of the machinery but they had to learn to adjust it guided by their son's behavior. Sometimes Mario and his parents were videotaped so that they could observe themselves with their child. Mario was tested many times throughout the program in order to get a more accurate reading of his hearing ability and to keep track of changes.

Mario's parents felt comfortable with their decision. Even in the early months when they were not at all sure the program would work for Mario, they felt that the attempt at natural speech was worthwhile. Since Mario's hearing problem was discovered so early, they felt they had a choice of communication methods. They wanted to exercise that choice to make his disability handicap him as little as possible. Sign language may be a good communication system for many and it may be the only communication system for children who do not get early sound and language stimulation. But if they have a choice most parents would choose natural language.

Auditory stimulation and speech reading can work. As Mario grew older he was enrolled in a special preschool group for hearing-handicapped children. This particular group was made up half of hearing-impaired children and half of normal-hearing children. This early exposure to normal-hearing children was supposed to be an incentive for Mario to continue his talking. A certain amount of Mario's understanding of speech was the result of improved hearing ability after his parents had worked very hard with him for some years. His comprehension also increased when he could see the person talking to him. One day when Mario was five, his mother was helping out at the preschool and she saw her son talking with a hearing boy.

HEARING BOY: Gimme the b'ue car.

MARIO: Not b'ue. It's bLue—bLLLLue. You can't even talk right. So there.

The work had been worth it. All that stimulation had paid off. Not only could Mario understand, he could criticize.

The basic principle of Mario's treatment (as of Brenda's) was to give him the sound that he could not have heard naturally and, since the sound was not perfect, give him plenty of it. This was done at a time when Mario was primed to build his own language with the building blocks made up of the language around him. Mario's parents could take pride in making it possible for nature to perform for their son the same mysterious miracle it did for everyone else: build a language. Mario's hearing became a bit worse, but he was able to go to school with normal children and hold his own. He continues with speech therapy every once in a while to maintain a consistent clarity in his speech.

Manual approach better in some cases. Is the verbal method best for all hearing impaired? Leah was a baby who got off to a bad start. She was premature and did not thrive the first half of her life. The doctor did not discover any specific illness, but Leah had a series of infections and fevers and was sick more times than she was well the first year. She did not develop the skills of sitting alone and crawling at the expected age but started crawling at about a year and started walking at two years. It was not until the second year, after her multiple health problems had cleared up to some extent, that her lack of speech became noticeable. Leah's parents came to realize that their child was slow. She continued to develop skills in walking and climbing between the ages of two and three. She also became more skillful at manipulating things and could assemble simple jigsaw puzzles. But she still was not talking. She did not seem to know her name nor did she respond appropriately to simple questions. She was learning most things at her slow rate but did not seem to be learning speech at all, neither understanding nor talking. Leah's parents took her to a diagnostic center at the university hospital near their home. They wanted to determine the best kindergarten placement for Leah. A hearing test was included in the routine child developmental testing. It showed that Leah had a moderate to severe hearing loss. The mystery of Leah's uneven development was solved: she was slow, but her failure to develop language was due to her inability to hear it. Early in her life Leah had medical problems; then she seemed to have motor problems. A hearing difficulty, which is not so obvious, is easily overlooked when parents, teachers and doctors are distracted by all the other more immediate problems. Not only was time lost for Leah, but her other difficulties had to be taken into consideration when choosing the best approach to communication.

Most children learn to talk without being taught. A child of normal intelligence just seems to pick up talking without anyone making any particular effort. Conscientious parents may enhance the learning process. Even neglected children, however, manage to learn. For a slightly retarded child like Leah, learning to speak doesn't just happen. Such a child must be taught and requires extra effort from parents and teachers. The verbal type of communication with amplification relies on the natural capacity of children to learn on their own. In the case of a hard-of-hearing child who has a general difficulty in learning (including learning sound), normal speaking and amplified hearing may not be a realistic goal. When Leah's parents considered these factors—developmental delay, intellectual disability and loss of the critical language learning period—they decided that Leah should be taught a form of sign language. They would learn to communicate with their child manually. By starting early and working with her they hoped they could help her overcome some of the limitations of this method.

Acquired Hearing Loss

Those born with perfect hearing can run into hearing problems later in childhood. There are many ways children can damage their ears. Childhood diseases such as German measles, mumps and chicken pox can leave a child with a permanent hearing loss long after the disease itself has passed. If your child has a serious illness, especially one with a high fever (the fever itself can be a hearing danger), you should have the hearing checked. Even if your child is already speaking you cannot be sure there is not a hearing loss just because you weren't told. The loss may be in only certain pitches and your child may not notice. Sometimes a child can suffer a blow to the head, damaging the middle ear. A common punishment for children in the last century was boxing them on the ears. One can only speculate on the amount of damage done this way.

Before Learning to Talk

If your baby becomes deafened or hearing impaired before learning to talk, your child will face many of the same speech and language learning difficulties of the congenitally hard of hearing. The further along your child is in language development before losing hearing the better. But even a child with fully developed speech and language will suffer if hearing or part of hearing is lost. Parents should be alert to possible dangerous conditions. Viral diseases contracted by the child can result in impaired hearing. These include the so-called childhood diseases and influenzas. There are vaccines for mumps, measles and rubella, and so these heretofore unavoidable illnesses of childhood can be completely avoided. Chicken pox is still around, but it never was as dangerous. The virus of scarlet fever seems to have weakened over the past few decades and so does not present the danger it used to. If, however, your child has a high fever from any cause, the possibility of hearing loss should not be overlooked. Ear infections and allergies can cause temporary conductive hearing losses. These middle ear infections and congestions can turn into permanent conductive hearing losses if left untreated. A temporary difficulty in hearing speech sound accurately during the speech learning period can have a permanent effect on your child's speech. Your child will reproduce imperfectly the sounds heard and by the time hearing has returned will continue the imperfect sound out of habit.

Your child is less likely to be exposed to dangerously loud sound in the early years, but in today's world we are all being subjected to loud noise. Too much loud noise wears out the hair cells in the inner ear so that they no longer respond to sound waves properly. Children injured in accidents can have their hearing damaged, especially those children who have sustained head wounds.

Sometimes the medicine used in the treatment of an illness will endanger your child's hearing. Some antibiotics, especially the streptomycin family, endanger hearing. Diuretics (drugs to relieve water retention) and antimalarial drugs can also be harmful. If an anesthetic was used during the delivery of your baby, it could cause a hearing loss, but it is usually temporary. Aspirin in large doses lessens hearing acuity.

These risk factors can seem pretty frightening, but though they can cause hearing loss their effects are not inevitable. You may want to have your child or baby's hearing checked or you may want to observe your child for response to sound. Parents are able to observe their child over a period of time and thus get a better idea about the child's response to sounds than a professional audiologist who sees the child only once.

From Exposure to Loud Sound

The following case may seem unlikely, but it is not uncommon: a self-induced hearing loss.

Timothy at twelve years knew what he wanted to be in life: a rock musician. He would listen for hours to his favorite groups. At first he would play records on his stereo in his room which was equipped with large powerful speakers. Timothy's family were driven to distraction by the sound. Although they did not appreciate rock music, they supported his interest in music and they did not want to discourage him. So they compromised by giving him a fine set of earphones through which he could listen all day to his music as loud as he wished without disturbing the rest of the household. The sound that the family had been disturbed by was about as loud as a heavy truck. Now Timothy was subjecting his ears to sound as loud as a jet plane at point-blank range. You may have heard of the deafness caused by too much artillery fire or the loud noise in factories. But music? Yes. Listening to traditional nonamplified music will not harm hearing, but if you amplify it enough electronically you risk developing a hearing loss.

Timothy went to every rock concert that came to town and listened raptly from the front row. He did not notice that the musicians he so admired were often wearing bulky earmuffs. At fifteen he started his own group with some of his high school friends. They found room in the school building they could use for practice sessions in the evenings. That year in a school hearing screening program, Timothy failed to hear certain pitches. The examiner told him he should avoid exposure to loud noise because the particular patterns of missed sounds showed the beginning of acoustic trauma or hearing loss from loud sound. The examiner went on to tell him that if he didn't change his listening habits his hearing would become worse. At first Timothy was shaken—a musician must be able to hear. On the other hand *he* didn't notice any problems. He knew he could hear as well as ever. The hearing screening must be wrong. So he continued as before. Naturally he felt it was better not to tell his parents about his screening. No sense in getting them all upset. His loss, which had started with being unable to hear one very high note, began to spread. Meanwhile he continued to listen to records through his headset, continued to attend rock concerts and continued to play and practice with his own group. One day he added a xylophonist to the group. Timothy tried the new instrument himself, but found that the upper notes weren't working. He could not understand what was wrong with the xylophone. He hit the notes harder. Still no sound. Finally the xylophone owner stopped him before he broke the instrument. There was nothing wrong with the xylophone; Timothy realized that he had lost even more of his hearing. Truly frightened, he went back to the hearing examiner for a complete audiological examination. He had lost some of the upper register of his hearing range. Timothy took immediate measures to protect his ears from the assault of loud sounds so that his hearing would not get any worse. He turned down the sound on the stereo and wore ear-protecting earmuffs. Unfortunately there was no way to regain the hearing that had already been lost. He could still communicate speech that was understandable because most speech is in the lower registers. He had to listen more carefully than the rest of us, however, because certain words we hear as different sounded the same to Timothy. Deaf and deft, shoot and suit are word pairs he can differentiate only in context. The tragedy is that certain subtleties of music are forever lost to this talented young man. If, in his maturity, he became interested in classical music, he would not be able to hear many of the rich overtones of the violin. Timothy, a youngster who treasured sound, will live the rest of his life in an impoverished sound environment.[7]

7. Some specialists think that presbycusis (the sensorineural hearing loss that occurs with age) results from a lifelong exposure to sound. Some people, however, do not lose their hearing, while others in similar sound environments do. There are probably other stronger factors such as heredity, even if long-term environmental sound trauma is a factor at all.

Safeguarding Your Child's Hearing

If you have a child, especially a teenager, you should be aware of some dangers to normal hearing especially for boys. Many people are not aware of the dangers of amplified music. Good stereo systems have more power than is safe to listen to if played at full volume. Because the fidelity is improved if the system is not driven to its maximum, the extra power should not be used so that the fidelity in the middle range of the available power will be sharper.

Another danger to hearing is riding on an unmuffled motorcycle. Encourage your child to have it properly muffled, not only to safeguard hearing but to comply with many communities' noise abatement laws. Your child may be earning money doing yard work. Long exposure to unmuffled power mowers can endanger hearing as well as exposure to using gasoline-powered chain saws. These are particularly dangerous because the person using them is right next to them and the danger increases the nearer the source of the sound. These three factors comprise the danger from acoustic trauma: loudness of the sound, nearness to the source of the sound, and length of time of exposure. Cutting one limb with a very loud chain saw may not be as dangerous as spending the whole afternoon with a loud (but not as loud as the chain saw) mower.

Intermittent Hearing Loss

Six-year-old LaVonna is starting second grade in the fall. Her parents are worried because of her erratic behavior during her first year at school. She started out very enthusiastically. The teacher reported that she was doing very well, was very attentive and was a model student. Toward the middle of the year, LaVonna changed. She simply did not pay attention in class. The teacher said she was not exactly disobedient or rebellious, just in a world of her own, often ignoring requests and dreamily going about her own way. Yet occasionally LaVonna would become her old alert and responsive self. The teacher, worried that there might be some problem at home causing her curious responses, called LaVonna's mother for a conference and found that her erratic behavior at home puzzled the family as much as her erratic behavior in school puzzled the teacher.

LaVonna had a slight lisp and was being treated by the school speech clinician to improve her S sounds. The speech clinician also noticed that some days the girl would be sharp and responsive, giving the impression that the lisp would clear up in short order, and on other days the therapy sessions would get nowhere. La-Vonna was not sick one day during the school year, but as spring came her chronic sniffle from allergies got worse. She never had a fever, but she seemed always to have a postnasal drip. During the years before school LaVonna had been ill several times with ear-aches, but all this was behind her now. At the hearing and speech screening at the beginning of first grade, LaVonna passed the hearing test and the lisp had been found by the examiner.

During a routine checkup LaVonna's mother mentioned her allergies to the physician. Luckily, as it happened, the appointment happened to fall on one of LaVonna's off days. The doctor found that the child's tonsils, which were visible, were enlarged and figured that the adenoids, which are at the back of the nose and not visible, were equally as large. The doctor also saw that LaVonna's nose was congested and that her ears looked stopped up. The doctor tested LaVonna's hearing on an audiometer and found that she had a moderate hearing loss. The hearing loss was worse some days and better other days. Sometimes LaVonna's hearing was fine, as it was on the day of the school hearing screening. If she had really seemed sick, the teacher and her parents might have worried about it or at least considered the child's hearing to have been impaired, thus causing her dreamy behavior. But without an earache to alert them, the parents and teachers never considered hearing loss. A few days after the medical examination LaVonna was sent to a specialist in ear, nose and throat disorders. A minor operation, a myringotomy, was performed in the office in the course of which LaVonna's eardrum was punctured (under anesthesia) and the middle ear was drained. Tiny plastic tubes, thinner than spaghetti, were inserted to keep LaVonna's ears draining. The doctor then started treating her allergy to clear up the congestion. Afterward, even when LaVonna's nose did get stopped up, she had no trouble hearing so she was able to pay attention and be her old self. The doctor thought it might be necessary to remove LaVonna's adenoids to enhance draining, but preferred to wait to make sure it was absolutely indicated. LaVonna's parents were surprised at the doctor's reluctance to take out the tonsils and adenoids, remembering their own childhood when everybody had tonsils and adenoids removed. Doctors are more conservative nowadays about removing tonsils and adenoids. It is felt that these structures have a function in protecting the nose and throat region from infection and reducing allergic reactions. LaVonna remarked to her mother one day a few weeks later that she often used to feel she was under water like a fish. She never feels that way now. She started second grade, the lisp cleared up, and she became a model pupil every day.

Conditions Making Hearing Loss More Likely

Someone once asked me if I thought every child should be tested for hearing before entering school. Yes, but I want to see this testing done much earlier. I would like to see every baby tested for hearing before going home from the hospital. At the present this is not deemed feasible because of the expense, but expense rarely seems to be a factor in other aspects of hospital care. More important, the tests are not yet reliable enough to accurately discern significant hearing losses in children to make the effort worthwhile. Some professionals feel that the rarity of hearing loss does not justify testing every baby. Other countries have infant testing programs, most notably Israel. This is an area in which a great deal of technological research is being done. There are many devices being tried, and perhaps within the very near future there will be a reliable and inexpensive method of determining whether or not your baby has a hearing loss before you leave the hospital. I hope such a method will become widespread.[8]

You should be alert to the various factors which could make your child more or more likely to suffer hearing loss. Any child with one or more of these conditions should be examined for hearing as soon as possible.

8. Most infant screening systems depend upon sensitive observation of the baby's reactions to sounds. For a newborn it would be ideal if a passive testing system could be developed. There is the technique of acoustic impedance measurement which measures the eardrum's resistance to a sound wave, which can be done on a sleeping infant. This is for middle ear function and health; hearing loss would be inferred rather than directly measured. There is another new technique of passive testing, auditory brainstem response (ABR). The air is stimulated with a sound, and electrodes placed on the scalp record the electric signals to the brain.

Hereditary Factors

It is estimated that about 50 percent of hearing loss at birth is hereditary. If there are others in your family who have had hearing problems since birth or later-developing hearing problems from an inborn condition, your baby would be in a high-risk category. There are towns and communities in the United States with a higher than normal population of hearing handicapped. There have been reports of whole islands where there is a large population of hearing-impaired people. It is easier to trace heredity in islands and isolated communities. Such communities contain a certain amount of intermarriage and so some inherited traits will show up more often than they would in the general population. When you evaluate the hearing of your family members, do not include the deafness which comes with old age. That, too, may be inherited, but it is not a problem during childhood or youth. If you have a family member who has had a hearing difficulty since childhood, inform your child's doctor of this condition, as it might relate to your child.

If there is anyone in your family who has had a cleft palate or cleft lip or any abnormality of the facial region, you may want to investigate your child's hearing.

Birth Defects

Some babies are born with certain deformities of the outer ear. Some of them have no significance to hearing, but others might be a sign of structural defects in the hearing parts of the ear. Sometimes birth defects come in groups of conditions, called syndromes. Hearing loss may thus be part of the group which could include mental retardation, blindness, kidney problems, heart problems, and albinism (lack of pigmentation). If a child has one of these syndromes there is a possibility that the hearing loss will be overlooked while everyone concentrates on the more obvious and visible conditions. Children with multiple handicaps are more difficult to test because it is not so obvious from such a child's outward behavior whether he was hearing normally.

If your child has any facial deformity there is a possibility of hearing loss. This includes clefts of the lip or palate or bifid uvula (if the drop-shaped flesh at the back of the mouth is divided in two).

If there is any abnormality of the ear seen through otoscopic examination (the instrument a doctor uses to look into the ear), there may be a hearing loss.

Conditions Before and During Birth

If you had any viral infection in the first third of your pregnancy your baby might be left with a hearing disability. The virus is especially harmful to rapidly developing tissue. In the first few weeks the inner ear is going through its most rapid development and is therefore most vulnerable. In the later periods of pregnancy the outer and middle ear go through rapid growth, making them more vulnerable. Malformations of the outer and middle ear are more easily remedied. The difficulty is that the infection may have been so mild that you barely noticed it and it may have occurred before you realized you were pregnant. Rubella (German measles) is the most well-known dangerous prenatal infection to a baby's hearing. But rubeola (red measles), chicken pox, influenza and other viral diseases you might have caught while pregnant can put your baby in a high-risk category. These diseases put the patient who contracts them at a risk of hearing loss as an aftereffect.

Rh incompatibility is another contributing factor in hearing problems for a baby. If the mother's blood and the baby's blood are incompatible there is a possibility of the baby's becoming jaundiced (yellow complexioned) after birth. A jaundiced baby is in distress and has a higher than normal probability of hearing loss.

Drugs taken during pregnancy are another danger to your baby's hearing. Thalidomide was the most famous of the damaging drugs taken by pregnant women. Other drugs are known to endanger the child's hearing if taken by the pregnant mother. These same drugs can cause hearing loss in the patient: the streptomycin family of antibiotics, diuretics and antimalarial drugs. You should not take any drug during pregnancy, even a nonprescription drug, without your doctor's consultation. And even if you think you might be pregnant or are trying to conceive, you should avoid drugs. If you are on medication prescribed by another doctor started before the pregnancy, inform the physician caring for you during pregnancy. Sometimes medical conditions make it necessary to take risks, but you should be aware of the risks. As for the so-called recreational drugs, there has been no scientific proof that they cause hearing loss. But I would not wait for scientific proof and would avoid them all while pregnant. Any drug taken by a pregnant woman is carried by the placenta to the baby.

Smoking in itself does not cause hearing loss, but it has been shown to be related to low birth weight. Birth weight of 1500 grams (3.3 pounds) or less puts a baby in a high-risk category for possible hearing loss.

Prematurity can also put a baby in a high-risk category. A baby is considered premature if it is born weighing under five pounds. In many cases of premature birth, the delivery is abnormal and the baby is injured or deprived of oxygen during delivery. Prematurity can also mean that the baby is not fully developed for life outside the uterus.

A difficult delivery for any reason should alert you to the possibility of hearing impairment. The birth process can cause physical injury to the baby's head and ears, resulting in hearing loss. You may not be aware of all the medical details of your child's delivery, but you do know whether or not it was more difficult than normal.

One sign of distress would be if your baby was cyanotic (blue complexioned). It is a visible sign of lack of oxygen. If your baby was starved for oxygen long enough to change skin color due to breathing difficulties, or any other reason, the baby would be a high-risk baby and possibly the condition could affect the infant's hearing.

How Does a Hearing-Impaired Child Act?
What to Look For

Sometimes a child will have none of the risk factors mentioned and still have trouble hearing. The parents should observe the baby or child carefully to uncover a possible hearing loss.

Does your six-month-old baby turn to sound or noises? At this age the baby should show awareness of your presence before you are in sight by the sound of your footsteps or voice. This is not a one-time test. Occasionally your baby might ignore you or not give an obvious sign of hearing you. As a parent, however, you can determine the customary behavior of your baby. If your baby never or only occasionally responds to hearing you before seeing you, be alert to the possibility of hearing problems. Does a sudden loud noise startle your six-month-old? Does the same unexpected noise make both you and your baby jump? Watch your baby's response to noisemaking toys. See if your baby is interested in the toy when it is hidden from view as you make it make its noise. You can use different types of noisemakers: little bells, click beetles, rattles, two wooden blocks hitting each other, crumpling cellophane (the stiff kind). Besides telling you whether your child is hearing, these games played with a normal hearing baby acquaint your youngster with different sound sensations.

Does your year-old baby try to imitate some of your speech sounds and syllables after you? If you say *baa* do you get a pretty good imitation back from the baby? Do you hear some attempts to say a few words such as *mama* or *dada*? Does your baby look at you when you call its name? If your child at one does all of these things, in all likelihood there is enough hearing for the baby to learn to talk.

At eighteen months your baby should demonstrate understanding of simple statements and commands such as "Grandpa is at the door" and "Get your coat" by going to the door or bringing the coat. If your eighteen-month-old baby does not seem to be responsive to any simple requests, you should be alert to the possibility of hearing problems or any of several developmental problems.

Does your preschooler always respond when called? Do you have to physically touch your child to get attention? Do you sometimes think that your child is not paying attention to you? All children are unresponsive at times, but if your child is usually unresponsive, there may be a hearing loss. Is it very difficult for a stranger to judge your child's responses to what is going on? One child may be very outgoing and give strong enthusiastic reactions to surrounding events. Another child may be quieter, more inhibited, given to very cool reactions. You know your child better than anyone else. It is you who must make the decision to see the audiologist based upon your assessment of your child's need.

How Severe Is the Hearing Loss?

If you take your child to an audiologist and a hearing loss is discovered you will be given an idea of the severity of the loss by the following descriptive terms: mild, moderate, severe and profound. In the mild range, your child has some difficulty hearing normal speech and misses whispered speech. The sound of a bubbling stream would probably be inaudible. The ticking of a loud watch might be just barely audible. In the moderate hearing loss your child finds loud speech hard to hear. Air conditioners and crying babies might also be hard to hear in this range. If your child is diagnosed as having a severe hearing loss only amplified speech is audible. Telephones, pianos and most machinery would not be heard by a child with a loss in the severe range. A profound hearing loss means that your child requires extreme amplification or an alternative method of communication. Heavy trucks, loud machines and airplanes are inaudible to such a child. Because of the nature of sound perception, these descriptive terms are more meaningful than the percentages sometimes given to express degrees of hearing loss. If your doctor or audiologist gives you a percentage ask for a translation to this descriptive scale.[9]

What You Can Do for Your Hearing-Handicapped Child

Talking to Your Child

At any level of handicap, your efforts are responsible in the main for your child's progress and opportunities for as normal a life as possible. Whatever the degree of hearing handicap, you must keep talking to your child. Your child needs more not less sound. Because it will be hard for your child to understand talking you should provide more of it. Repeat what you say if you do not think your child has picked up your message the first time. Do not wait for your child to indicate that you were not heard. You and your child can listen to the world together. Many sounds that you hear you take for granted—the roar of the car engine or the sound of rain on the roof—but your child may not hear them at first. Or your child may actually be able to hear them but they sound much

9. Sound intensity is measured in decibels (dB). O dB is the normal threshold; 110 dB would be loud enough to be painful. Frequency (pitch or tone) is shown in cycles per second or Hertz (Hz). An audiogram shows the threshold in dB or the softest audible sound heard by the patient for each of the frequencies (250, 500, 1000, 2000, 4000, 6000, 8000Hz). The significant frequency range for speech is 500 to 2000 Hz. It should be noted that O dB is not total silence but an average threshold determined experimentally. Many people hear sounds softer than O dB. Total silence cannot be measured in dB (the mathematics goes haywire with total silence).

softer than they do to you. If sounds are faint and difficult to hear we have a tendency to ignore them as being too much trouble to attend to.

> YOU: It's starting to rain.
> YOUR CHILD: Rain?
> YOU: Listen—it goes duh duh duh duh duh [opening window].
> Now you can really hear it! DUH DUH DUH DUH.
> YOUR CHILD: I hear it! I'm wet too.
> YOU [closing window]: Hear it now? Duh duh duh?
> YOUR CHILD: Yeeah. On the roof. Duh duh duh.

Your child has some hearing, but it takes effort and practice on both your parts to make use of it.

Talk to your child in a face-to-face position. In this way many children with mild to moderate hearing losses can automatically pick up some speech reading. You can see how it works with the following experiment. Turn down the volume on your TV set so that you hear nothing. You won't be able to follow the speech on the program even though you can see the speaker. Then turn up the volume to the point you are just aware of the sound and turn off the picture: you still won't be able to follow the speech. Now, without increasing the volume, turn the picture back on. By looking as well as listening with greater concentration than you are used to giving TV, you will be able to understand better what is going on because you are using two senses instead of one. If your child needs help in comprehension give speech reading a chance to develop.

If your child has a permanent hearing loss you will need professional guidance. You will have to provide your child more stimulation to learn language than the ordinary amount most children receive. You can learn how to help your child at the speech and hearing clinic. There you can meet other parents with hearing-handicapped children and share experiences with them. If your child has a hearing aid you will need instruction on caring for it and adjusting it. If your child needs manual language, you will need to learn this new language yourself.

Hearing Aids

Should your child have to have a hearing aid, you will need to be under the care of a professional audiologist certified by the

American Speech-Language-Hearing Association. In many places it is legal to have a child fitted with a hearing aid merely by the person who sells these devices who may or may not have some training in hearing disorders. These people are in business to sell hearing aids not the treatment and training of the hearing impaired. They often need a release from a medical doctor before they can sell the hearing aid, but there is no requirement that they follow up and counsel on the use of the aid. You especially need the services of an ASHA certified audiologist with a baby or young child. The audiologist will have kept up with the latest in research on hearing disorders and hearing aids. Each year there are improvements in the state of the art. Your audiologist will keep retesting your child to note and adjust the electronic equipment to changes in hearing. The audiologist understands language development and comprehension, which is more complex than merely being aware of noise.

Communication

Your audiologist can help you in your decision of what kind of communication your child should learn. Do you want to try the auditory-oral route or the manual route? The auditory-oral method will take more time and effort from you and your child, but if successful your child will be able to live in the society of normal adults. The manual route may be easier for you and your child, and your child may develop other talents without being burdened by the task of learning to talk. There are fine and interesting people in the society of deaf people who communicate manually and many seem to lead satisfying lives within it. But it is still a limitation. The decision is not to be made by professionals alone. They have not only the professional expertise to provide the necessary information but a personal philosophy and a realistic assessment of you the parents' own abilities and resources. But you have to decide if you can accept your child's wearing a hearing aid, and if you can learn to operate it and teach your child to do so. Some parents are ashamed of the hearing aid and won't put it on their child when going out in public. On the other hand, can you accept gesture language? There are people who are repelled by seeing others communicate by sign language. How do you feel? It does no good to decide how you *ought* to feel. Whatever technique and philosophy you accept eventually you must be honest with yourself at the beginning.

Different Educational Settings

After you have made the choice about which method of communication your child should learn, you must make decisions about what kind of school setting your child should be placed in. Again, even with professional guidance, you know your child better than anyone else and are in the best position to decide what is right educationally and evaluate the child's progress.

Preschool years. During the preschool years you can choose to keep your child home all the time. If such a service is available, you can have a clinician visit you periodically at home to treat your child and advise you in familiar surroundings. Another arrangement would be for you and your child to visit a clinic periodically for instruction. You could also enroll your child in a preschool group for hearing-impaired children which might or might not be integrated with hearing children. If you are lucky enough to live in a community where there is a home demonstration program, this might be the preferred arrangement for the preschool years. There is even a correspondence course for parents with deaf and hard-of-hearing children. See Organizations for Further Information, p. 259 for the name and address.

School years. At six years or the beginning of school age, you will have to decide on your child's educational setting. Your earlier decisions will have had some bearing on your child's educational opportunities at this point. There is the residential school for the deaf run by most states, and there are now special day schools for the deaf and hard of hearing. In the day school your child would live at home but get instruction tailored to the special needs of the hearing handicapped. There is also the possibility of the special class within the regular school. The academic instruction would be in special classes, but the lunch and playground activities would be spent with normal-hearing boys and girls. This experience would help your child to get along in the normal-hearing world. Another approach would be mainstreaming: your child would attend classes in the local school with normal-hearing children. The teacher would be alert to your child's special problem but the class would be a regular class. If your child has sufficient communication skills, this is the most desirable arrangement. Your child would not only learn the same things as everyone else did right along with them, but would be forced to maintain normal forms of communication. You must determine whether your child's skills are up to this type of setting.

Higher education. If your child has gone to school in an integrated setting with normal-hearing children, any college would be appropriate depending upon your child's interests and academic skills. The college or university advisers may have to ask the professors to make certain adjustments for your child and it may be necessary to select courses carefully. If, on the other hand, your child has been mostly with other hearing-impaired children and uses manual language more than speech, you might consider the one college in the U.S. for the deaf, Gallaudet in Washington, D.C. Here higher learning can be pursued in American Sign Language.

The Future for the Hearing Handicapped

There is a link between the growth of the technological wonders we all enjoy and the attempt to provide delivery of sound to the hearing impaired. Over a hundred years ago, Alexander Graham Bell, a teacher of the deaf, worked at inventing a hearing aid. This primitive attempt at a hearing aid was soon seen to have much wider reaching uses and was soon developed by Bell into the telephone. But it wasn't until the transistor that hearing aids became powerful enough to enable the infant and child born with a hearing impairment to learn language in the natural way. Before the transistor, hearing aids were more useful for those who had already learned to talk before losing hearing. I think there will be enormous changes in the treatment of hearing disabilities in the future. Perhaps there will be more powerful hearing aids with greater fidelity which can be engineered with the precision to compensate for the individual's specific type of hearing loss. Perhaps we will see electronic prosthetic devices surgically implanted. Perhaps microsurgery will enable doctors to repair inner ear structures. Since hearing treatment is changing, parents must be aggressive in finding out what is available and what is best for their child.

Suggestions for Parents of Hearing-Impaired Children

- Don't assume that your child's hearing is all right just because you notice response to loud noises.
- Have your child tested or screened for hearing if you have any doubts about your child's hearing or the child falls into a high-risk hearing loss category.
- Find out about your child's hearing as soon as possible. Don't wait until a "better" age for testing hearing.
- If you find that your child has impaired hearing talk more not less.
- Get professional help as soon as you learn of the hearing loss.
- If your child is not attempting any speech at two years old, check for hearing loss.
- Don't ignore an earache in your child.
- Do not assume that your hearing-impaired child cannot learn to speak.
- Be aware that your hearing-impaired child will have to work very hard to learn to speak.
- Explore using hearing aids even for a tiny baby.
- If your child needs sign language, become fluent in sign language yourself.
- With any form of communication, make sure your child is paying attention before you speak or sign. Be in a face-to-face position.
- Be careful to conserve your child's hearing by seeking prompt medical treatment for ear infections and discouraging long exposure to loud amplification: motorcycles, chain saws, blasting stereos, and so forth.
- Be aware that nasal congestion can cause a temporary hearing loss, from a cold or hay fever. This hearing loss can interfere with learning.

5

How to Help Your Child Produce Clear, Articulate Speech

Mispronunciations Often Heard in Children's Speech

Five-year-old Becky says *wabbit* instead of *rabbit* and *wed* when she means *red*. Becky's parents are concerned, but her kindergarten teacher is not surprised, having often heard the W/R mistake. It is not unusual for a child to misform one or more sounds, the most troublesome of which are S, Z, K, J, SH, L, TH and R. These sounds are even more difficult when they are combined in words such as "*cr*ack," "*cl*am," "*scr*ape," "*spr*inkle," "fou*rth*" and "six" (si*cks*). Confusion of S and Z and SH is so common that it has its own name, lisping, a word that those afflicted with a lisp cannot pronounce.

How did Becky get this *wed* for *red,* the W pronunciation for all her R words? It is not found in the speech of the members of

Becky's family, so it seems a mystery to them how she could have picked it up. The fact is that when Becky was just learning to talk three years ago there were *many* sounds she couldn't say. Her parents were so delighted that she was trying to communicate by talking at all that they weren't too fussy about how clear a word had to be in order for them to understand it. Becky might have said *'poon* while waving a spoon in the air. Her mother was more interested in *what* the baby was saying than *how* she was saying it, and understood. Seeing her handling the spoon helped her understanding.

Many babies replace a sound they can't make with one they can make, as in *wabbit* for *rabbit*. Sometimes they leave it out altogether: *'ed* instead of *red*. Occasionally the baby's attempt at the unsayable sound will result in a sound so weird that the alphabet fails to describe it. If the child is young enough we accept the misformed words and usually don't correct them. We don't expect babies to make every sound come out right the first try.

What Is Talking?

Unconscious Movements We Make When Speaking

I used to ask people what they thought they were doing when they talked. The usual response was that they thought very carefully about what they were saying. But I would ask again what did they *do* to make the words come out? When the person realized that I was not asking about the content of the speech but the production of the speech, the response was usually an exasperated shrug of the shoulders. The reply was usually "I just open my mouth and the words come out." "By magic?" I would ask. My point would gradually become apparent to the by-now confused person I was questioning (usually a student) and the typical answer would be "Probably I move my mouth in certain ways." This person forgot that we do anything at all when we speak. We take talking for granted, but it is really very hard to do. Think of what you have to go through, for instance, to say the word *shoe* (a relatively simple word). You have to hump the middle of your tongue toward (but not actually touching) the roof of your mouth, at the same time pursing your lips slightly, and holding the sides of your tongue against your back teeth to form an airtight seal. You must control your breath so that just the right amount of air is forced between your tongue and the back of your front teeth. Meanwhile the back of your tongue must be raised to shape the vowel OO. In addition to all this, you have to do it very fast and be prepared to go on to the next set of sounds which will be just as complicated but different. If you think about what you are doing when you are talking you will forget what you are trying to say. If you could see an X-ray movie of all that goes on when you are talking, you would be amazed that anybody can do it at all.

Of all the animal species on the earth, we are the only creatures who can talk. Some birds can make sounds which imitate talk but by using a different physiological system. Many animals communicate, and there may be an argument about whether or not their communication system is language, but no one thinks that their communication system includes speech. Just what is speech anyway?

Speech Is Meaningful Sound

Any sound you can hear needs a source of vibration to set the pressure waves in air going, a source of energy to set the vibrator going and some kind of resonator to amplify the sound enough to carry it to your ears. The human being, like many other animals, is equipped with soundmaking ability. The outgoing breath stream is the energy source to start the vibrations. The vibrator is the larynx (voice box), where there are two folds of flesh which reduce the size of the opening from the lungs to the throat when they are almost closed. You can find your own larynx by touching the front of your neck while saying *aaah* and feeling the vibration. The exhaled air forces the two folds to vibrate, producing the vocal tone. This is the same principle as stretching a blade of grass between your thumbs and blowing through it. If you do it right you will get a high-pitched tone. The bones of the head and the mouth and nose cavities act as the resonator. Resonators usually amplify or increase some parts of the produced sound while damping out other parts of the tone, resulting in the particular character of the sound. For comparison, think of a violin. The string is the vibrator, the bow (or the arm of the violinist) is the energy source, and the wooden case is the resonator. In the case of the trumpet, the mouthpiece is the vibrator (in combination with the lips of the trumpeter), the lungs of the trumpeter provide the energy, and the tube and bell of the instrument make up the resonator. The reason that the same note played on the trumpet and the violin sound so different is that the resonators are so different, which illustrates how much a sound can be changed by changing the shape of the resonator. The human being can change the shape of the resonator by lifting the tongue and opening the jaw and changing the shape of the lips. This is easy to demonstrate. Using the same tone of voice say *aaah* then *eeeee* then *oooooo*. The change you hear is the change of resonance. If you watch yourself in the mirror you can see how your mouth changes shape between these vowel sounds. While most of the sound energy of speech is during the vowel sounds, it is the consonants which make speech articulate and understandable. Each time you say a vowel (there are about fifteen vowel sounds—not letters—in American English) you have said a syllable. By modifying the breath stream between syllable centers (vowels) in certain ways you create the consonant sounds. In general the consonant sounds are made by impeding the breath stream totally or partially by constricting some part of the vocal tube (the speech apparatus from the larynx to the lips), resulting in a noise. A noise is a nonmusical, nonharmonic sound such as a clap or air escaping a tire. For instance the S is made by lifting the tip of your tongue to the roof of your mouth behind your front teeth close enough to make the exhaled breath hiss but not tight enough to stop it altogether. If you stopped the breath stream altogether in that position and then released it the result would be a T. So to simplify a complicated process, the sound of speech is made by the exhaled breath activating the larynx. This exhaled breath comes in bursts, one burst to a syllable, and each syllable is made up of a vowel tone formed by sizing and shaping the mouth. Each syllable may have a noisy beginning and/or end, the noises or consonant sounds made by constricting the breath stream at some point. These consonant sounds are briefer in duration and are more difficult for children to learn than the vowels. Therefore they are most likely to be formed poorly by children as they are learning to talk. The remarkable thing about speech is its speed. While you are talking, your tongue, lips and soft palate (the moving articulators) are moving constantly against your teeth and hard palate (the fixed articulators) with a precision unmatched by any other skill you have or could acquire. But rather than being merely a virtuoso feat, your speech conveys meaning.

The different speech sounds are grouped in syllables and the syllables either by themselves or in combination make up words. The words make up sentences and go together in certain ways to convey meaning. So not only does a child need to know how to form the individual vowels and consonants, but must put them in a particular order to express words. The words have to be chosen, and also the grammatical arrangement of the words must be learned. All this is before you figure out *what* you want to say. All of this is automatic for most people; not only don't they have to think about what they are doing, they mostly are unable to think about it.

Is Mispronunciation Normal?

Becky's parents understand that her mistakes in talking are not unusual but are still concerned whether they are normal. The truth is that mistakes *are* a normal part of the learning process. In fact some mistakes are inevitable during some stage of a child's speech learning. No child will give up using a word merely because a sound in that word hasn't been perfected. But as children get older we expect them to refine their pronunciation so that it becomes more like the speech of the people around them. When this happens we realize that the child has outgrown baby talk.

Becky's problem with pronouncing her sounds is the most common speech problem in children. Three to 6 percent of children have speech disorders, and of these children 80 percent have trouble speaking clearly.[1] We describe these problems as mumbled speech, lazy tongue, thick speech, lisp, baby talk, but they are all basically articulation problems: difficulty in forming and pronouncing the sounds of speech. An English-speaking child should be able to pronounce all the sounds of English by first grade. By the end of first grade a child should be able to pronounce all or almost all the sound combinations (SN in *snow*, PL in *play* etc.). If

1. C. Van Riper, *Speech Correction: Principles and Methods*, 6th ed. (Englewood Cliffs, NJ: Prentice-Hall), 1978, p. 156.

L. D. McDermott, "The Effect of Duplicated and Unduplicated Child Count on Prevalence of Speech-Impaired Children," *Language Speech and Hearing in the Schools*, vol. XII, no. 2.

In an effort to evaluate two methods of counting prevalence of speech disorders in school, these percentages were found. I have rounded the numbers to the nearest percentage point. The data on prevalence of speech disorders vary widely, depending on the investigator's criterion of speech disorder.

your child is not talking plainly after starting school, you should be alert to the possibility that speech will not clear up on its own but will need help.[2]

You might not want to wait until school age to see whether your child's speech is developing normally. Some speech sounds are easier to produce than others. Therefore your child is more likely to say the easier sounds at an earlier age than the more complicated sounds. Sometimes the hard sounds are hard because they are more difficult to hear, such as the TH in *thin*. For other sounds the necessary movements are complicated and exacting as in the case with the S in *see* or the CH in *chin*. There are also some sounds which occur so infrequently that your child doesn't have much chance to hear them or to practice them such as the ZH in "television."

By four years of age your child should have mastered all the easy sounds which include all the vowels and the following consonants:[3] N as in *new*, M as in *my*, P as in *pig*, Y as in *yellow*, H as in *horse*, NG as in *sing*, D as in *do*, F as in *fish*, W as in *wait*, B as in *boy*, G as in *girl*, C as in *cow*, and T as in *two*. If your four-year-old has trouble saying any of these, you might be concerned about speech. On the other hand there are a number of sounds your four-year-old might not say which should not worry you. These are the sounds we expect to be mastered later in the child's speech learning period, often developing after four years. These include the TH in *there*, as well as the TH in *thin* (two different sounds), the R in *rabbit*, V as in *violin*, SH as in *shoe*, CH as in *chin*, L as in *lady*, J as in *joy*, Z as in *zoo* and S as in *see*. Even if your child at four mispronounced all of these sounds, the child could still be considered to be progressing normally.

Helping a Child Overcome Normal Mistakes

Three-year-old Sam says "Wook at de witto pish." Sam's mother can translate it right away as "Look at the little fish." Sam's

2. L. D. Shriberg, "Developmental Phonological Disorders," in *Introduction to Communication Disorders* (Englewood Cliffs, NJ: Prentice-Hall, 1980), p. 290. In a survey by Hull (1971), 2 percent of the children in the United States were found to have extremely deviant articulation—a more stringent requirement than I would make for an articulation survey.

3. Ibid., pp. 270–271. The sounds your four-year-old should have mastered are based upon a study by E. Prather, D. Hedreck and C. Kern. These developmental norms were based upon speech of a large number of children two to four years old.

mother might ask, is Sam's speech normal? Yes, Sam's speech is normal for his age even though it is full of mistakes. If he were five years old it would not be normal. Sam's speech will clear up considerably in the next two years, but it can't be guaranteed to do so.[4] Then Sam's mother asks, "Suppose his speech doesn't clear up by the age of five? Will we regret not starting a speech program for him at the age of three?" The dilemma is that we believe that the earlier we start to treat Sam (if he has a speech disorder) the better our chances of success will be, but we have no way of telling the difference between children who are making mistakes due to the normal learning process and those whose speech will not clear up by itself.

Sam's parents don't have to decide whether or not Sam has a speech problem in order to help him with his speech. If there is no disorder, Sam is merely developing slower than his parents would wish, and if he lives in good speech learning surroundings, his baby talk patterns should disappear. Sam's parents will be anxious to provide as rich and as nourishing a speech environment as they can.

On the other hand, Sam's parents may be *too* understanding. Sam has taught his parents *his* dialect or speaking style so they are more likely to understand him than others who do not spend as much time with him. Sam should talk to his grandparents or other relatives. His desire to be understood should inspire him to be as clear as possible. He may be sloppy with his parents because he realizes unconsciously that they have a forgiving ear. Yet, there is a line between being too understanding and being rigid or punitive about a child's speech. Sam's parents can do as much harm by being too demanding and overcorrecting his speech as they can by being too understanding. Sam's mother is helping him in the following conversation by providing a model for the correct pronunciation. Notice how she repeats the troublesome words, prolonging and emphasizing the problem sounds. By lengthening the F and L sounds in the words Sam's mother gives him a longer time to hear them.

4. Ibid., p. 289. A procedure for predicting whether or not a child's speech will clear up without treatment would be very useful. Speech researchers are working on a method now. Many clinicians use factors such as how easily the child can imitate the trouble sound and how often the sound mistake occurs. But so far, I am not completely satisfied with available prediction measures.

SAM: Wook at de witto pish.

MOTHER: Look at the what ffffffffffish?

SAM: Witto fffpish.

MOTHER: Oh you mean the lllllllllllllllittle fffffish. Llllllet's see how many llllllittle fffffffishes there are.

SAM: Pour pish.

MOTHER: Hmm, I see one ffffish, two fffish, three ffffish, ffffour ffffish.

SAM: Fffffour fffpish.

MOTHER: Let's count them together to make sure. [The two count them in unison.]

How is this conversation helping Sam's speech? First it is non-punitive. Instead of saying "Don't say witto, say little" or "Don't say pish, say fish," Sam's mother carried on a positive conversation which supplied Sam with the correct models of his mispronounced words. Second, Sam's mother realized that the F in *fish* was easier than the L in *little* because she heard an attempt at the F but not the L and so backed off from the L's and concentrated on the F's. She also understood that *fffpish* was progress toward the correct pronunciation even though it was not perfect. It was true that the wrong P had not disappeared, but the correct F had appeared. Children often keep the old mistakes right next to the new correct pronunciation for a while. The P in *pish* (*fish*) had become a habit and was hard to drop right away. When the two of them were talking together, something that most children enjoy, Sam was able to hear his mother and himself at the same time and he had a chance to compare the two. Sam didn't know consciously that he was having a speech lesson, but he was learning a new talking pattern. He didn't learn it completely in a few minutes and he will revert to the old pattern many times. More sessions or conversations with mother and/or father, to give Sam extra exposure to the sounds he can't pronounce and time to say them back, may be all Sam needs to help him along in his speech. Many parents do things like this without realizing that they are giving their child a speech lesson. We all have a natural tendency to emphasize sounds as we talk with our children, just as we have a natural tendency to name things around us to our baby or small child. Sam's parents can also become aware of his particular speech difficulties with these little "lessons," as they will be listening to him more closely. Conversations such as the one between Sam and his mother ideally are short and frequent and fit naturally into everyday activities.

Finding the Mistakes

You may have a preschool child whose speech is not always clear, but you may not be able to tell right off exactly which sounds are wrong. Sam's mother seemed to find the precise mistakes Sam was making. You can find mistakes too but not all at once. Listen to your child's speech and every time you hear a word that sounds funny, say to yourself: "Why does it sound wrong?" You can imitate your child's pronunciation out loud and compare it to your pronunciation and the difference should be obvious in your ear and in your mouth. Then you can use that word in conversation several times, emphasizing and prolonging the problem sound. If you can help your child clear up mispronounced speech without the child ever realizing that the speech was not right in the first place, you have helped in the most natural and desirable way. In this way your child need never become mouth conscious and have to worry about how to talk as well as what to say. For example:

YOUR CHILD: See my new toos?

YOU: New what?

YOUR CHILD: New *toos* [pointing downward to the new shoes]?

YOU [thinking]: Hmm. Toos instead of shoes. Let's see, toos—shoes. What's the difference? Oh, the beginning there is a T instead of a SH. . . . Anything else wrong? Shoes—toos. No, the rest of the word seems OK. I must remember to listen to other SH words.

Later:

YOU: Look at the pretty sea shell.

YOUR CHILD: Sea tell?

YOU: Yes, sea shshshshshshshell. I found it on the beach. Put it to your ear. It says shshshshshsh [you demonstrate].

YOUR CHILD [listening to the shell]: I hear it!

YOU: Is it saying shshshshshsh?

YOUR CHILD: Yes, it says shshshshshsh.

YOU: That's right, the sea shell says shshshshsh like I do when I want you to be real quiet.

YOUR CHILD: [giggling]: The sea shshshshell says "Be quiet."

You don't expect the SH sound to be magically corrected after this conversation, but it is a beginning. No child wakes up one morning resolved to give up the baby way of saying SH. If your child is getting the hang of the SH sound in words, you will hear it said correctly some of the time and incorrectly at other times. You know there is progress when your child moves from only occasionally pronouncing the SH in words correctly to the correct pronunciation half the time and then to only occasionally mispronouncing it over a period of months.

Sound Games

If you are able to identify the sounds your child misforms you can play games with them. Don't make them parts of words or letters of the alphabet. Give them personalities or make them into what some creature says. They can become auditory toys. For instance, Sammy Snake goes "sssssssssssssss" and scares people. Timmy Tick Tock lives in the clock and says "tuh tuh tuh tuh." The motor boat goes "puhpuhpuhpuh." When the cat gets angry it says "ffffffffffff." When you are singing a song and have forgotten the words you go "la la la la." When there is a mosquito in your room at night you can't fall asleep because it says "vvvvvvvvvvvvvv" (high pitched). The bees in the garden say "zzzzzzzzzzz" to tell you to keep away. For example you could play a game with your child.

> YOU: Who am I? I say "Zzzzzzzzzz."
> YOUR CHILD: A car?
> YOU: Nooo, I live in the garden. "Zzzzzzzzzzzz."
> YOUR CHILD: A flower?
> YOU: No, but I like flowers. "Zzzzzzzzz."
> YOUR CHILD: A bee! You're a bee?
> YOU: You be a bee too. What do you say?
> YOUR CHILD: "Thththhzzzthth?"
> YOU: Let's both be bees.
> YOU AND YOUR CHILD TOGETHER: "Zzzzzzzzz."
> YOU: Be an angry bee.
> YOUR CHILD: [scowling]: Zzzzzzzzz!

Once these identities are established, you can take up the game any time anywhere—at lunch, in the car, waiting on line at the check-out. Your child may think these are just fun noises, but all these noises are sounds that are used in words. Imitating the angry cat is not the same as pronouncing the F in *fish* or *fan* or *laugh* correctly, but it is a beginning. You can make a game of the sounds without making your child self-conscious about pronouncing words.

Causes

Are Mispronunciation Problems Physical?

Tongue-tied? Becky's parents remain worried about her speech even though the kindergarten teacher seems untroubled by the W/R confusion for a five-year-old. They speak plainly to her, helping her pronounce sounds she has trouble with in a positive way, but they think that the problem might be physical. Could there be something wrong in Becky's mouth? Of course there could be some problem in her mouth, but I have found physical causes to be less common than people think. Could she be tongue-tied? How could parents know? What is "tongue-tied" anyway? Becky's parents could play a follow-the-leader game with her. Father opens his mouth in a big yawn. Becky does the same thing. Keeping his mouth wide open, her father lifts his tongue to the roof of his mouth (he practiced beforehand in the mirror). Can Becky do this? She may not be able to do it on the first try, but if she can do it after a few attempts, she is not tongue-tied. Mother tries another follow-the-leader game. "Let's touch our noses with our tongues," she says. If Becky shakes her head, her mother says, "I can't either, but this is the way I try. See how far you can get." If Becky can raise her tongue outside her mouth she is not tongue-tied.

There is a little piece of connecting flesh from the underside of the tongue to the bottom of the mouth. You can find it by feeling with your finger under your tongue toward the back. If this piece of flesh is too heavy, is placed too far forward or is too short, it is thought that the movement of the tongue will be restricted or "tied." There are certain sounds where the tongue must be lifted— L, S, Z, D, N and T—and therefore impossible to say if the tongue is truly tied. Parents suspecting that their child is tongue-tied can go to a surgeon and have the flesh (frenum) clipped. They are generally disappointed, however, to find that the operation does not cure the speech problem. Even if the tied tongue were the problem and the child had truly been unable to place it properly for the tongue-lifted sounds, the operation would not be an immediate cure. The child would still have to *learn* to lift the tongue for those sounds and break the old pre-operation tongue placement habits. The current professional opinion on this matter is that surgery is mostly unnecessary. In almost all cases of an apparently restricted tongue, the child can learn acceptable speech without surgery. It could be that the frenum seems tight because the child has not tried to stretch it by lifting the tongue. Since any surgery for speech improvement must be followed by speech therapy (to learn the new movements made possible with the surgery), it is advisable to try speech therapy without surgery first, avoiding risk of infection and some pain.

Tongue too big? Becky's parents may wonder if her tongue is too big for her mouth. Many children with poor speech seem to have enormous tongues. It is thought that even if a newborn baby could learn to speak, speech would be impossible because the tongue is so large in relation to the mouth cavity that there is not enough room for the tongue mobility necessary for speech. As children grow older however the mouth enlarges more than the tongue. Sometimes with children of Becky's age it seems there is not enough room for the tongue to move. But looks are deceiving. The tongue is an especially difficult organ to measure. It appears larger when it is relaxed than when it is tensed. If Becky's tongue is never tensed enough for clear speech—and clear speech takes a pretty athletic tongue—it will appear too large to her parents. Thus a large-looking tongue may be the result rather than the cause of unclear speech. It cannot be shown that tongue size within the normal variation of human anatomy has any relation to skill in speaking. There are some inborn deformities which can include an enlarged and blunt tongue affecting speech, as in Down's syndrome (see Chapter 3). I, however, am not convinced that it is the size in these cases as much as the impairment of nervous system function which causes speech problems.[5]

Cleft palate? Becky's parents can dismiss immediately a cleft palate as a cause of their daughter's speech problems. A cleft palate is apparent at birth and is not something that is acquired later

5. J. E. Bernthal and N. W. Bankson, *Articulation Disorders* (Englewood Cliffs, NJ: Prentice-Hall, 1981). In 1941 McEnery and Gaines recommended against surgery for clipping the lingual frenum. Most authorities still agree with this opinion. McEnery and Gaines also investigated the relationship between size of tongue and speech. They did not find tongue size to be a factor in speech problems. Bernthal and Bankson, however, say it has not been adequately investigated.

in life. Chapter 6 gives more information on the cleft palate. There are so-called acquired clefts from injuries to the roof of the mouth, but they are not true clefts. If these injuries are serious enough there might be some trouble speaking, but you would know of such an injury. This type of wound can occur when a child falls while sucking on a lollipop with a hard stick. You can prevent this from ever happening by limiting your children to suckers with soft loops.

Missing teeth? Besides noticing the *wed/red* problem, Becky's parents notice that she is saying *thoap* instead of *soap*. Since she has just begun to lose her baby teeth, they think they have hit upon an explanation. Common sense tells you that you need teeth to make an S. Some children, however, have contradicted common sense and everything I know about how speech sounds are formed. I saw a child who had lost his upper front teeth and his lower front teeth at once and simply had a hole in the front of his mouth. His S's were perfect. I don't know how he did it. I would have thought it to be impossible. He must have naturally changed his way of speaking to compensate for the missing teeth. Now if one child can speak perfectly with so many teeth missing, it cannot be inevitable that missing teeth cause speech problems. Therefore when we see missing teeth in a person with a speech problem we cannot assume that the missing teeth are the cause. The boy with the missing teeth may have been an exceptionally talented speaker. There are cases in which the missing teeth may contribute to speaking diffi- culties in a child. Still, I am convinced it is not so much what you have in your mouth but what you do with it that causes good or poor speech.[6]

Is Poor Hearing Causing Mispronunciation?

Could it be that Becky doesn't hear the difference between *thoap* and *soap* or *wed* and *red?* Becky's parents would find it hard to believe that she can't hear the difference between these

6. Ibid., p. 122. Studies on large numbers of children show that the incidence of sound errors, particularly *s*, *sh* and *f* in children with missing teeth is higher than in children whose teeth are intact. Some children do, however, pronounce their *s*, *sh* and *f* correctly in spite of their missing teeth.

sounds.[7] Her hearing had been checked during the hearing screening at her kindergarten. The parents were told that Becky had enough hearing ability to develop speech normally. Becky's parents were especially relieved that they did not have to worry about poor hearing acuity as a possible cause of poor speech. Becky went through a couple of bad winters of colds and earaches. She received excellent medical treatment for her ear infections but was never given a hearing test at the time. Becky's parents may not realize that when she was sick she probably did not hear well. Even though the infection has been cured, the temporary hearing loss Becky suffered could have been the start of her talking difficulties even though the hearing is completely restored by now. She may have been in the process of mastering the R and S sounds when suddenly her hearing dimmed so that all sounds seemed muffled to her. She could hear the sounds she already knew because she knew what she was supposed to be hearing. If you lose some of your hearing ability suddenly from a cold or hay fever, you can manage to understand others because you know what you are supposed to hear. But it is possible that Becky had not completely learned either to hear or to say the R and the S sounds in words. Speech learning doesn't take a vacation during sickness, so she may well have learned the muffled (to her) sounds. The mistakes can continue after the earache has been cured and hearing restored because Becky got used to hearing and saying the sounds wrong. The mistakes became a hard-to-break habit.[8]

Is Careless Listening the Problem?

What Becky's parents may not realize is that although she hears the difference between the S and TH, W and R, that differ-

7. L. D. Shriberg, "Developmental Phonological Disorders," in *Introduction to Communication Disorders* (Englewood Cliffs, NJ: Prentice-Hall, 1980). It is not known when children tell the difference between speech sounds they hear. F. D. Eimas, E. R. Sigueland, P. Jusczyk and J. Vigorita reported in 1971 that infants of a few months can tell the difference between consonants B and hard G. Most speech pathologists believe that sound discrimination and sound production are connected. If Becky overgeneralizes her TH and S producing *thoap* for *soap*, why not the other way around? She never says S for TH (*sirty* for *thirty*).

8. J. A. Carrell, *Disorders of Articulation* (Englewood Cliffs, NJ: Prentice-Hall, 1968), p. 52. A clear explanation of how a temporary hearing loss can lead to a permanent speech problem, persisting long after the hearing loss has been cleared up.

ence may not be important to her. If you think about the word
blouse you may remember that you have heard it pronounced
with a Z at the end sometimes and at other times you have heard it
said with an S (like a hiss) sound at the end. Since the difference
did not change the meaning you ignored it even though you could
hear it. The problem with the TH and S sounds is that though
Becky can hear the difference, she doesn't bother to separate them
in her mind because the substitution of the TH for the S doesn't
cause much confusion in meaning.

To find out if Becky does hear the difference, her parents can
play some word games. Mother shows Becky a picture of a child in
bed who doesn't look well (sick) and another picture of a heavy
rope (thick) and asks which is sick. She also tries a picture of a
mouth and a picture of a mouse. In this way she can tell if Becky
hears the difference between the S and the TH sounds when that
difference is important to understanding the meaning of the word.
Another game is Tell-me-if-I-say-it-wrong. Here is one way the
game can be played. Father says "We drive the car down the
woad. Let's eat some wice." Becky will have the delightful task of
telling her father he is wrong when he says *woad* or *wice*. She can
hear the difference between *rice* and *wice*, *woad* and *road* if she
can point an accusing finger at her parent's mistakes in speech. On
the other hand Becky's parents may find out through their games
with her that although she hears the difference between *mouth*
and *mouse*, she doesn't pick it up between *thoap* and *soap*. Maybe
Becky will differentiate between the TH and S when the difference in sound makes a difference in meaning. But if the difference
doesn't change the meaning, she won't bother with it.

None of us bothers to listen for differences in speech sounds
when these differences do not change our understanding of what is
being said. It is not that we are all lazy. There are so many sounds
coming into our ears at such a great rate that it is remarkable that
we can understand and process speech at all. Therefore it is not
surprising that we ignore small variations in speech sounds when
they do not help our understanding of what is being said. *Thoap*
and *soap* mean the same thing to Becky, so there is no need for her
to listen to the difference. *Mouth* and *mouse* mean different
things, so it is necessary for her to notice the difference if she
wants to understand what is being said. Her understanding of *sick*
and *thick* also requires this differentiation. We rarely listen to sin-

gle words by themselves. Usually the words are embedded in a sentence so that whether or not you listen for the difference between *sick* and *thick* the intended word is obvious by the rest of the sentence. Moreover, the difference Becky listens for in other people's speech between TH and S is the first step in learning to listen for that same difference in her own speech (apparently a more difficult task).

Inconsistent Mispronunciation

Since Becky's parents have been listening closely to her speech, they have noticed that she sometimes says *thoap* instead of *soap* but sometimes it is *toap* instead of *soap* and a couple of times it was *soap*. They were pleased enough to hear *soap* but wonder if the new mistake they heard is cause for alarm. No, it is cause for joy. She is breaking a bad speech habit. They say that practice makes perfect, and nothing is harder to correct than something you practiced wrong, not only for hours and days but for years. Speech is like that. The reason Becky started saying *wed* for *red* is ancient history. Today she says *wed* for *red* because that is what she said yesterday. Each time she makes the mistake the habit becomes more deeply ingrained. If Becky's way of attempting the word *soap* or *red* starts to change even to a new mistake, her parents should be pleased that the habit is getting weaker. Any weakening of a mistaken speech habit is a good sign. If *thoap* changes to *toap*, we know it is changeable and has a better chance of changing to *soap*.

Many parents concerned about their children's speech notice a surprising thing: some words are said correctly and other words seem stubbornly incorrect. If they listen and analyze carefully they discover that the difficult new words are more likely to be pronounced correctly than the old familiar standbys.[9] Take the problem of TH at the end of words. Many children say *baf* instead of *bath*, *wif* instead of *with* and *toof* instead of *tooth*. It would seem that these children cannot make their mouths form TH at the end

9. J. A. Carrell, op. cit., p. 33. Early learned movements provide the basis of habits. But unlike walking, in which a misstep results in a fall, a mispronunciation does not have any such consequence. Moreover, if the mispronounced word is understood it communicates as well as the correctly pronounced word. These incorrect patterns become embedded in a level beneath consciousness and therefore are harder to change.

of words. But when the parents listen more closely they find their children pronounce *earth, path,* telephone *booth* and *fourth* perfectly. They do not say *earf, paf, boof* and *fourf* as you would think. How come? At the early time in their lives that the children learned the words *bath, with, tooth,* they could not manage that TH at the end of words and so made do with the closest sound that they found they could pronounce—F. Because these words were learned early, they were learned well and they were learned wrong. The habit of saying *baf* instead of *bath* has gone on a long time. By the time the children have learned the words *earth, path, booth* and *fourth* their mouths had matured enough to handle the TH at the end. Moreover since these words had not been part of their vocabulary at all, they did not have the pattern of mispronouncing them and had no bad habits to overcome so were able to say them correctly from the beginning. Yet the old habitually mispronounced words remain mispronounced. This is another example of how habits of long standing are strong and resistant to change. And also how much easier it is to learn something completely new than to replace something you already know with something else.

Can a Child Acquire a Speech Problem from Family or Friends?

Becky's parents aren't satisfied yet. They may understand why her speech continues the way it is but are still looking for a specific cause that started it as well as ways to correct it. Could Becky have picked up her way of pronouncing words from another child? Becky's parents have noted that several of her playmates make similar mistakes in speaking. Are speech defects contagious? It depends from whom. Unlike chicken pox, you can't pick up a speech disorder from just anybody. It is extremely unlikely that Becky could pick up or catch a speech problem from another child unless the circumstances were very unusual. The child with poor speech would have to supply most of the speech that Becky heard, more than the speech from her family, other adults and other children who speak well. Moreover, this child would have to be a person Becky looked up to and wanted to emulate. On the other hand if it were Becky's father or mother who said *wed* instead of *red* and *thoap* for *soap* she might well have caught it.[10]

Kevin was brought to my clinic because he mispronounced so many words that his speech was difficult to understand for a boy of seven. Other children at school made fun of him. Among other mistakes he would say *tumb* for *thumb* and *ti'en* for *chicken*. Second grade was an agony for him, and he began to speak less and less. A teacher's aide brought him to the clinic to supplement his speech lessons at school. He was quite willing to work in therapy and seemed to do well in his time with us. But we were disappointed at his progress. Between sessions he seemed to forget everything he had learned. We set up an appointment with Kevin's mother. Her first words of greeting, "A wu Mi' Bara?" (Are you Mrs. Barach?), solved the mystery of Kevin's lack of progress. Kevin's and our work was being undermined at home. Kevin talked exactly like his mother. His mother's way of talking did not reinforce lessons so laboriously learned in school and in the clinic. In fact it had the opposite effect. The cause of Kevin's speech disorder was now clear. His speech learning was fine; it was just that the particular speech he had learned so well was not correct to most people. At first it was hard to get Kevin's mother to understand that Kevin really had a speech problem. After all, to her ears he sounded fine. She finally admitted that she was not sure of her own speech skills and had all her life been timid about talking to people. She was not sure she wanted to change her own speech, but if we felt it would help her son she was willing to try. So we put mother and son on the clinic schedule and gave them plenty of practice to do at home. They could help each other. Kevin's speech cleared up after a few months of therapy. His mother's did not progress so quickly. Her speech did not become really perfect and perhaps it never will be, but it is greatly improved. Her improvement was necessary for Kevin's cure. Kevin caught his speech from his mother the way we all catch our speech from our mothers. Unfortunately the speech Kevin caught was not regularly accepted speech.

10. Ibid., p. 36. The author discusses the possibility of twins inventing their own language. Although many authorities discuss the possibility, there has only been one documented case of this. It was widely publicized. But further investigation of the invented language revealed that it was a variation of English and not a whole new language—just a peculiar dialect. I am sure that twins reinforce each other's pronunciation errors.

Can Parents Affect the Natural Timetable of Development?

Becky's parents wonder if Becky's speech difficulty could be part of her psychological or developmental makeup. Although Becky did sit up at eight months and walk at sixteen months (more or less the normal time according to the pediatrician), she did not seem at the time to be doing these things as early as the children of some of their friends. Becky did say her first word at eighteen months and began stringing words together into sentences at two and a half years. These speech milestones are within normal limits but not precocious. Pronouncing her words correctly could be one of the things she is a bit slow in doing. But will she catch up eventually?

It is true that each child has a unique timetable of development. The norms that are so widely publicized are merely averages. If the average age at which a baby sits up at first is seven months, that does not mean that five months or nine months is an abnormal time for a baby to sit up. And it does not mean that seven months is the best time for a child to first sit up. Most five-year-olds have mastered all the speech sounds. But some normal five-year-olds have not mastered the R and S sounds—they are still working on them. Parents may understand this, but it is not as easy to accept a timetable on the slow side of normal as it is to accept one on the fast side. It is always so reassuring to see the developmental milestones—walking, talking, running—as they are achieved by your child. Even though Becky may be a perfectly normal little girl on a slower timetable, it is understandable that her parents may be anxious during the interim between the average time children develop perfect speech and the time *she* develops it.[11]

Becky's parents must make sure to provide her with the optimum conditions for developing her speech sounds in every way they can. They must realize that her rate of development can be slowed down by uncaring, unstimulating conditions or advanced by

11. A. H. Hayden, R. K. Smith, C. S. von Hippel, and S. Baer, *Mainstreaming Preschoolers: Children with Learning Disabilities* (Washington, D.C.: U.S. Government Printing Office, 1978). This introduction to a chart of normal development cautions the parents not to expect too strict adherence to the norms. Children not only develop at different rates but develop skills in different orders. Moreover, the children's experiences also influence their development.

loving, encouraging conditions. The following is an example of speech-inhibiting conditions.

Tad's speech problem is not being helped by the parents and is probably being aggravated. The scene is at the dinner table, the child has speech like Becky's.

> TAD: Gueth what I thaw today.
>
> MOTHER [to father]: Did you get the car fixed?
>
> TAD: It wa' a weally . . .
>
> FATHER: Eat more, talk less. No. The guys at the garage still can't find the rattle.
>
> TAD: You should have theen it. It . . .
>
> MOTHER: I guess the Harrisons will be moving out soon. [To Tad]: Stop that pouting and eat your dinner.
>
> TAD: It wa' thomething . . .
>
> FATHER: Don't talk with your mouth full—can't this child talk straight for a change?
>
> MOTHER: Stop playing with your food.
>
> TAD [to himself]: I hate taters, I hate cawwots. I hate evewything. [Continues to spread mashed potatoes in a thin sheet over the plate.]

Tad is desperate for attention and wants to communicate. His parents are elaborately avoiding listening to him. When they finally do notice him, it is to scold him for pouting, table manners and bad speech. It is unlikely that Tad could have done anything right in this situation except to withdraw. All his overt behavior was criticized. Speech is overt behavior, and a child needs practice to learn it. It is true that grownups have rights too and need time for adult conversation, but Tad needs conversation too.

To see if Becky's parents are hindering her speech development, they should be asking themselves some important questions. Does Becky have enough opportunity to talk? Do we seem to want to hear what she has to say? Is the talking atmosphere relaxed? If Becky is tense or anxious, is she likely to revert to a more juvenile talking pattern?

Can Emotional Problems Cause Good Speech to Deteriorate?

Parents have often noticed that when their child is anxious about something, the first sign of the anxiety they see is that their child takes up thumb-sucking or another baby habit that had been

discarded years ago. By starting up old behaviors a child can return to a more comfortable time of life. If Becky acts the way she
did as a baby, maybe, she thinks, she will again get all that nice
treatment she had as a baby. The trouble is that now her parents
don't want to play her baby game. Her baby act doesn't evoke
their warm and loving attention. Becky's anxiety may not cause
her to pick up old habits but it may make her hold on to outmoded
habits such as saying *thoap* for *soap*.

Becky's parents should ask themselves whether she is going
through more than the usual emotional bruising of growing up.
Some anxiety on entering a new school is to be expected, but if the
anxiety were crippling or lasted over a period of months it might
be considered more than usual. Becky's parents should look into
their own family history. Certain events may be having an effect
on the little girl. It is often difficult for parents to judge how an
event affects a child from her direct reaction. If there were a
recent death in the family or if Becky's parents were having mari-
tal difficulties, Becky might be reacting by not continuing her
speech learning. Her speech could be a sign of inner turmoil.
Becky's immature speech may be her own reaction to events out of
her control.

Becky's friend, four-year-old Lucille, seemed to be learning to
talk very well and then, suddenly, her speech changed. Could she
be forgetting the good speech she had already spoken? She who
had said "pussy cat" clearly two months ago was saying "puddy
tat." Worse, she was saying "Me likum puddy tat," when two
months ago she had said "I like the pussy cat." Her pronunciation
and her sentence structure seemed to be going backwards. Lucille's parents were surprised and worried that she was suffering
from some degenerative condition. They brought her to a speech
clinic. The clinicians were also surprised but not astonished. They
were very interested in everything that had happened in the past
few months around the time Lucille's parents had noticed the de-
terioration in her way of talking. There had been no traumatic
experience either physical or psychological which could explain it.
There were no deaths, divorces or moves in the family. The only
unusual event had been the birth of Lucille's brother three months
ago. Since all the other possible causes of the child's speech deteri-
oration had been ruled out, it seemed reasonable to consider her
reaction to the new baby, who had forced her to give up her

exclusive place in the family and have to share it with a newcom-
er. The speech clinicians talked with Lucille's parents and discovered that Lucille's speech was not really reverting back to old
discarded ways of talking. This so-called baby talk was a new
pattern that Lucille had never used before. It could have been
Lucille's idea of what baby talk should sound like. But why did she
talk this way? It could be that the new baby was a competitor for
the attention and affection of her parents and Lucille took an "if
you can't lick them join them" attitude. Lucille pretended to be a
baby too since that was the way to win the attention and affection
game. Now Lucille did not consciously figure all this out, but
when she saw all the fuss made over the new baby, she got the idea
that the way to get a fuss made over you is to be a baby. She knew
she couldn't be tiny again, but she could talk like a baby. As a bid
for attention it was pretty successful because she did cause her
parents to worry about *her*. They gave her attention when they
expressed their concern. Since the effect was desirable she kept it
up and the baby talk was reinforced.

If your child has been talking well and then the speech falls
apart and seems to be developing backwards, you should be concerned. Ask yourself if there has been an accident or illness which
has changed your child's abilities for talk in any way. If there has
been no such cause, look for some event which has changed your
child's life, some adjustment which had to be made. A new member of the family, a new baby, the remarriage of a parent, a death
or a move to a different house, a different school or a different city
may have this effect. Although you don't want to reinforce the
baby talk, realize the going backwards in learning to talk is a cry
for help. Your child needs you and the security of your love.

Lucille gradually dropped her fake baby talk when her parents
spent more time with her. They included her in the baby care and
were sure to praise her for grownup behavior such as helping with
household tasks (things the baby could not do). The baby became
Lucille's baby too. Now the baby has the problem of having two
"mothers" but Lucille talks fine.

Does Chronic Illness Affect Pronunciation?

Michael says "Wah doo, bu'o my too. Lee fo', o'en de do' " for
"One two buckle my shoe. Three four, open the door." Michael

had been born with a heart defect. He has been in the hospital many times and has had more operations than most of us have in a lifetime. In spite of all this he is a bright and active little boy with an astonishing vocabulary for a five-year-old, once you are able to understand his pronunciation. How could his medical problems affect his speech? His damaged heart does not affect his talk directly, but his medical condition puts him in an emotional and physical environment that is not normal. His parents are less demanding—they are thankful to see him alive—and the confined environment of the sickroom keeps him in surroundings somewhat like a baby's. Michael does not have independent mobility enjoyed by other children. He has made friends but they have been adults in various health care positions who have been tolerant of his speech. His life until a few months ago has been more like a protected baby's than a normal child's. It is not surprising that he acts immature for his age. He is less patient, less cooperative, less outgoing than the other children. He is particularly trying to the kindergarten teacher because he has not learned to wait for his turn. He is unwilling to share his own things and yet does not respect the property rights of others. He needs special help in his speech as well as patience and firmness in guiding his social behavior. His parents must make the same demands of him that they would make of a normal child.

How to Tell Language Disorders from Pronunciation Problems

Children with articulation disorders have trouble pronouncing their words because they have either not learned to move their mouths properly or have not learned to choose the appropriate sound for the word they want to say. Their problem is simply one of not forming the words correctly. There are speech disorders, however, which are language-forming problems. A child may have trouble putting the words together to say something meaningful. A child may not know enough words, or may not be able to change words by adding -ing or -ed to alter their meaning slightly. These are difficulties in basic language structure and often basic thinking structure. Children with language disorders, as they are called, generally have poor pronunciation in addition to the poor language structure. We don't know immediately when we hear a child who mispronounces words whether it is simply a matter of poorly formed speech sounds or poorly formed language. What we *hear* is mispronounced words. We must listen and decide whether the child would speak normally if the pronunciation were cleared up with vocabulary and grammar suitable for the child's age level. For example a child might say "Pu' de boog on de deth" for "Put the book on the desk." This seems to be a pronunciation problem as the words are correct and all there but said badly. If, however, the child said "Pu' uh deth" we would suspect more than a pronunciation problem. The words are said badly but also the child has left out any attempt at the article *the* and it is not clear that there was any attempt to say the word *book*. Whether we are parents or professionals, we ask whether the mispronunciation is a symptom of poorly learned language or merely what sounds like poorly learned mouth movements. (Chapter 3 describes this in detail.) If we hear speech which is way off the mark we suspect language-forming problems. Articulation disorders or sound-forming problems can be the whole communication problem or just one part of the communication problem.

A Multiple Communication Problem

Four-year-old Nancy says " 'Aw 'i' 'aw' " meaning "I saw a big dog." Nancy's mother is concerned because she knows Nancy's speech is not right for her age. Nancy's grandmother says she has a lazy tongue and her speech certainly sounds that way. Her speech cannot be understood even by her immediate family. Nancy, however, seems to understand other people. When one of her parents asks her to pick up her shoes, Nancy does so. Nancy's family therefore does not feel that she is unable to hear or to understand speech. If a four-year-old's speech is so far from the way it is supposed to sound that not even the forgiving and understanding ears of the parents can understand it, there is cause not only for concern but for immediate action. While Becky's parents might well wait for the school speech therapy program, Nancy's parents should not wait but seek help right away. School work, especially reading, is based upon speech skill. Nancy cannot learn what the letter *d* means in *dog* when she has not mastered the sound D in the spoken word *dog*. Also does Nancy's failure to use the plural S in *dogs* means that she cannot pronounce the final S or that she doesn't understand the concept of the plural? Arithmetic, which is based upon number concepts, requires language and thinking skills that Nancy's parents are not sure she has. It is unlikely that a child of four with such unclear speech would simply be delayed in her learning pronunciation timetable and would catch up if left to herself.[12] She may have trouble not only forming her words but finding the right words to form.

Helping a Child with a Language and Speech Disorder

Nancy's parents should find help for her now, but in the meantime they should be careful to talk to her slowly, carefully enunciating each word. Nancy in all likelihood will need therapy, and it is a good idea for her parents to develop the habit of giving their child concentrated attention. Nancy will have to learn to behave in the structured and spotlit environment of the clinic. The attention of her parents and the structure of games they play with her are good practice for this situation. A game Nancy's parent could play with her might be Do-what-I-do. The parent would do something with a set of blocks and Nancy would be asked to do the same thing. The next stage would be that the parent describe in simple terms what is being done with the blocks and then ask Nancy to describe what she is doing with the blocks. The block activities should be tasks which Nancy is able to do easily such as building a tower of four or five blocks or arranging them in a line. This kind of game is similar to many of the activities Nancy will encounter in therapy, and some practice will make her treatment go more smoothly. The particular game is less important than the practice of doing something with an adult.

The Older Child with an Articulation Problem

The Boy Who Did Not Outgrow Baby Talk

Many parents think that baby talk will be outgrown. There is no way for the parents of a five-year-old to predict whether or not

12. A. H. Hayden et al., op. cit. According to the chart of normal communication development, Nancy should be able to follow three interrelated commands in order. She understands *one* command, which is what one expects from a one- to two-year-old. At three she should have started plurals and pronouns and *-ed* endings. The use of plurals makes the distinction between one and more than one, which is the beginning of number concepts.

the pronunciation mistakes will clear up by themselves. In many cases all the child needs is a little more time than normal to refine and perfect speech pronunciation. There are cases, however, of children keeping speech mistakes way past the time that normal speech is expected. The older such a child is the more difficult it is to correct the speech.

Jack at ten says *wed* for *red* and *wabbit* for *rabbit*. He says some words with the S sound which don't come out right such as " 'Tay heoh" for "Stay here." His speech is not too different from Becky's. Everyone can understand him, but anyone listening to him realizes that there is something "off" about his way of talking. The cruel fact is that the same speech mistakes that are acceptable or even a little cute in five-year-old Becky sound ridiculous and jarring in ten-year-old Jack. The other children taunt him at school, imitating his baby talk and laughing at it. The adults around Jack may not be so overt in their cruelty but nonetheless display their disapproval. At home Jack's father is impatient every time Jack makes a mistake (almost every time he speaks) and makes remarks such as "Can't you ever say anything right?" Jack's mother winces visibly whenever he talks. Jack's teacher never calls on him to recite in class, feeling the less he has to talk the better. And in fact, Jack talks very little. He spends most of his time by himself or with his dog. The dog seems to be the only one who doesn't hate his talking.

The Disadvantage of Delaying Past the Critical Speech Learning Age

When Jack was five years old no one worried about his talking. Jack's family assumed he would grow out of his mispronunciations—when they noticed them at all. Now that he is ten they are not so sure. Jack's father's way of coping with his doubt is to blame Jack for being too stubborn or lazy to correct his pronunciation. Jack's mother is unsure what to do and so does nothing except show her distress. For whatever reason he failed to refine and perfect his speech, Jack needs help. He has been talking that way for years and his bad speech habits are much stronger than Becky's. In addition, Jack is past the age of learning speech sounds naturally. Until about the age of seven or eight, children are more pliable and open-minded in their learning of speech sounds. They can pick up a foreign language quickly and easily and come to speak it like a native, a task very difficult to do in later years. Jack now needs to unlearn old ways of talking and learn new ways. It will have to be a conscious effort rather than the unconscious learning done by younger children. If we could turn back the clock we would have advised Jack's parents to get help for him when he was five or six years old. But his speech can still be helped and his parents should get that help as soon as they can. They should also have counseling themselves so that they can understand their role in helping Jack clear up his speech and how their attitudes are affecting his speech.

Moreover, Jack's speech clinician will have to treat more than just his speech. Help will have to be given to undo the psychological damage from the years of teasing. Jack's shyness and tendency to withdraw from social activity grew out of his insecurity about his speech and also need to be overcome. Speaking correctly would be the start of Jack's building his self-confidence.

Help for Articulation Disorders

Becky and Michael and Kevin are children who are slow in learning to pronounce all the sounds in words. They may be on a somewhat slower timetable than others or there may be some external reason preventing normal development of their speech sounds. The poor speech model in Kevin's case and the immaturity brought on by Michael's sickroom life seem probable reasons. Whatever the reasons, will these children catch up on their own? Can the parents alone guide their children to better speech? Or will it be necessary for these children to have the specialized help of a speech pathologist? Should the parents wait until these children get to school so that the school speech clinician can help them? All of these children have pretty straightforward speech difficulties. They are called articulation disorders by speech pathologists. Articulation refers to the formation of speech sounds in words.

Advantages and Disadvantages of School Speech Remediation

Since Becky's, Michael's and Kevin's speech problems are very typical of speech problems of children in school, the speech therapy program in schools that offer one will most likely be equipped to handle them. Public school speech therapy is convenient and it is free. You don't have to take your child to a special place; the therapy is conducted in school. Because the surroundings are familiar, there is no need for the anxiety that often comes with going to a new place. The speech clinician will coordinate the speech program for your child with the regular school program. This provides a useful and natural medium for speech therapy and the opportunity for your child to use the new speech.

One disadvantage of school therapy, however, is that often it doesn't start until the second grade. This late start gives those children whose speech will clear up spontaneously a chance to improve on their own, even though earlier therapy would improve the chances of success for those who need extra help. A greater disadvantage is that you, the parents, are often removed from involvement. The teacher refers your youngster to the school clinician. If you are not assertive about being included or are unwilling to take the initiative in visiting school and talking with both the teacher and the speech pathologist, the whole treatment can proceed without you. And if you don't know what is happening in therapy, you are not in a position to be much help. Sometimes, as with the case of Kevin's mother, your active participation is not just desirable but necessary. Your child, like Michael, may need more from you than just speech help. But the exclusion of the parent is *not* inevitable—the teacher and the clinician do want your participation. They know that their job will go smoother and faster if they can get you to help. If you are willing and if you show interest, you can take as active a part in your child's school speech therapy as you want.

Finding Available Services

Investigate whether your school has a speech therapy program and how much time the speech pathologist can give to your child. Most school systems in the United States have some speech and hearing services as part of the regular school program. In general one speech specialist serves more than one school. If the speech pathologist can see your child (usually in a group) at least two periods a week, you have a good program available to your child at least in terms of frequency of contact. Some smaller school systems may not have enough clinicians to see each child twice a week and may only get to your child once a week or even less often. Effective speech therapy requires at least two sessions a week. Your child can receive extra help from you or the classroom teacher under the guidance of a professional speech pathologist. You can find out whether your school has speech therapy services by calling your local school superintendent or school board. They should have the information on the number of clinicians in the school system, how often the children are seen and at what age the children receive therapy. You don't have to have your child enrolled in school to obtain this information.

Since the passage of the Education of the Handicapped Act the responsibilities of the public school system in the United States have changed somewhat. Under the new law every child is entitled to whatever special education is needed for that child to achieve maximum academic potential. In order to qualify for these services your child would have to have a handicapping condition. If your child's speech is judged to be handicapping, your child falls into the population covered by the law and remedial services which include your active participation must be provided. In some communities the speech remediation is completely handled by the special education department. In other communities there is still a speech remediation program as part of the regular school program. The law is applied differently in different places, and the judgment of handicapping condition is different. For children with severe handicaps there is not a problem, but for those with mild disorders which might be outgrown there might not be services available as they would not qualify as handicapped. In such a case if you didn't want extra help for your child, you could investigate a special speech and hearing clinic or a speech pathologist in private practice. Chapter 9 gives more information on finding available speech and hearing services.

If you are sending or plan to send your child to a private or parochial school which does not include speech therapy as part of its program, it is still possible for you to get public school speech therapy for your child. The Education of the Handicapped Act applies to all children, not just those in public school. You will probably have to transport your child to the nearest public school which does offer speech therapy at the time it is being offered. This also holds true for those public schools which do not have speech therapy. Your child should go to the nearest school offering therapy for speech remediation services.

Evaluating the Services Your Child Receives

No matter what the setting for your child's speech treatment, you will want to know how well the treatment is going. How can you tell? First by listening. That is how you knew that your child had a problem in the first place. If you feel that you have become so accustomed to the way your child talks that you are not a good judge, ask a relative or friend less familiar with your child's speech patterns to listen for improvement. If you visit your child's speech teacher you can ask how many sounds were produced wrong when your child started and then at the end of the school year ask how many sounds were learned and which sounds were left to learn. Your child's clinician should be able to explain what was accomplished or why an objective was not accomplished. If you feel your child is not showing the improvement you had hoped for, ask the speech clinician for an explanation. If your expectation was unrealistic the clinician should explain this. If your child's case is more complex than you had thought, the speech clinician should be able to discuss this with you. You will be able to tell if the people treating your child are dedicated caring professionals if you talk with them.

Speech Therapy in Isolated Areas

There are some isolated areas where it is not practical for a speech pathologist to visit every child who needs help with speech every week. If you live in such a remote place you can set up long-distance therapy with the speech teacher in the nearest school. Some speech clinicians in the western states of the United States, where travel is difficult during the long winter, have set up programs for parents in which they give the parents instructions in how to help their child's speech after evaluating the child in person. They keep in touch with the parents by mail and recheck the child in person after a period of some months. This may not be the most desirable way to get speech therapy but it shows that cooperation is possible between parents and speech pathologists and together they can make a helping team.

Is It Possible to Have Too Much Speech Therapy?

Jack's parents were late in recognizing his speech problem. His life would have been happier if they had sought help for him at five or six. On the other hand can parents be too concerned too early about their child's speech? Before you rush your four-year-old to the nearest speech center, consider Will. Will is also ten years old and has been in speech therapy off and on since he was four. He not only had trouble with his R (*laddo* instead of *ladder*) and S but several other sounds as well, especially the sound blends such as in *street* and *crisp*, which he pronounced *weet* and *wip*. Will's parents were very worried about his speech and they gave him the opportunity not only to hear them make sounds he was having trouble with but to show him the mouth movements they used to make these sounds. They took every chance they could to help him with his speech. When he went to see Santa Claus at the store they helped him say Santa Claus instead of Tandy Caw. They took him to a speech pathologist and carefully drilled him between lessons. He learned the speech sounds all right, but his speech became more and more labored. He had left therapy by the time he started school, but the home drill continued. In the second grade the school speech clinician heard his speech during a routine speech screening and found it unusual. The word *street* was pronounced "sssssssssterrrrreetttttt" with two syllables. The clinician thought that he needed help, not realizing that he already had plenty of it. The more the speech clinician worked on Will's speech the more effortful it became. The school clinician talked with Will's parents and recommended that they take Will to the local speech clinic. The people at the clinic thought that Will's R was not quite right and found his SH as in *shoe* and *ship* to sound like S (*soe* and *sip*). Will was a model client. He put his all into speech therapy; his parents were model clinic parents and carefully drilled him each night. Still his R's were stubborn (*bwotho* instead of *brother*) and it seemed the harder he tried the stranger his speech became. He could tell you exactly the movements necessary to say *shoe* or R as in *Peter Rabbit*. He would think about what he was doing with his mouth as he talked. Finally one day the clinician at the clinic threw away the lesson and just talked to Will. They told each other riddles and silly jokes. Will got the giggles. He said "My brother told me this one. . . ." The clinician heard *brother* said right for the first time. "Your what?" the clinician said, hoping to hear the word said correctly again. Will froze and said "Mmmmmmy bew-rotho." He had become too mouth conscious. Tense because of all the attention to his speech, he was trying as hard as he could to talk right. But speech isn't like that. We expect it to flow smoothly and effortlessly. Having to think about it makes it not only more diffi-cult to speak but the result doesn't sound good. Will had been "overtherapied." The family, the teachers, friends and relatives had focused on Will's speech. Everyone was listening critically every time the child opened his mouth. There were no vacations from speech improvement. He worked longer and harder than anyone should have to work on his speech. His sister, who was one year younger, had started with the same difficulties as Will's but the parents never heard her mistakes because they were so busy listening to Will. Will's sister's speech cleared up by itself. Now what do I advise Will's parents? At ten years speech patterns don't change overnight. Will should be left alone about his speech. The parents should stop listening to him so critically. They should en-courage some new activity not related to speech such as sports or music. He should be given the opportunity to succeed at something else.

What can Will's and Jack's experiences teach parents? Mostly, that extremes are to be avoided. The best commonsense approach for parents to take is somewhere in the middle ground between too much help for their child and none at all. Help should be provided when it is needed, but the parents' help must aid the natural speech learning process instead of turning talking into an overin-tellectualized procedure.

Seeking Professional Help: What to Expect

If your child falls half a year or less behind these guidelines, extra stimulation from you may be all that is necessary to help in pro-nouncing words. If your child's speech is further than a half year behind you should consider a speech and language examination. You should have had your child screened for hearing long before; if not, a hearing examination would be a must. Chapter 4 has information on hearing testing for children.

Your child may seem to need more than the usual stimulation of speech at home and kindergarten to learn clear articulate speech. The pronunciation learning may be fine, but your expectations may not be realistic. If you are in doubt and feel you need help in determining whether or not your child is learning to pronounce words normally, the speech clinician can give you the information you need. If therapy is not necessary, your mind will be put at rest and you will have professional reassurance that your child is normal. If therapy *is* needed you can begin at a good speech-sound learning time of your child's life.

Analysis of Your Child's Speech

Whether you take your child to a speech clinic or wait for the school speech pathologist (or both) there are some things you and your child can expect from professional help. First, anyone who treats your child will have to find out how the youngster actually speaks: how each sound is produced (twenty-five consonant sounds and fifteen vowel sounds—not letters) at the beginning, middle and end of words. For instance your child may not be able to say TH at the end of *bath* and yet be able to say a word beginning with TH such as *thumb* correctly. It is necessary to find out *which* sounds are wrong, *how* they are wrong (what the child is doing instead) and *where* they are wrong. The clinician must understand the mistakes before they can be remedied. You as parents will be interested in the clinician's findings. You will learn whether or not they agree with your own ideas. You may soon be able to listen to your child's speech a little more analytically.

You Will Be Part of the Speech Treatment Program

During the therapy time you should keep track of what sounds are being taught in the clinic or school and listen for changes in pronunciation at home. The clinician may send homework back and/or explain what you can do to reinforce the speech lesson. For example the clinician may tell you, "Today we worked on listening to F words. Every time you find a word with the F sound in it you and your child can write it down in your notebook." Then at home when you see a fork you can add that to the F word list in the notebook. Soon you will find fish, fan, phone, leaf, roof, etc. You may also look through magazines and cut out pictures of F word objects. Most of the speech homework will be something you and your child will do together.

If you take your child to a speech clinic you may be invited to observe a session. The best way for you to see what is going on in therapy is through one-way glass, so that you can see into the therapy room but those in the therapy room cannot see you. If you have a preschool child, what you will see will look like games. The successful clinician will make the sessions enjoyable as well as therapeutic. A possible activity could be:

> CLINICIAN: Let's see what I have in my magic bag [holding up a bulging bag]. What things have our special sound? THTHTHTHTH [pulling out object] THimble, does this have our sound?
>
> CHILD [nods, smiles and raises hand but does not speak].
>
> CLINICIAN: Good. TH in THimble is our special sound. Now what's this? [pulling out plastic tooth]. TooTH—does this have our special sound?
>
> CHILD: Yes, I hear it.
>
> CLINICIAN: Good. Here's something else [holds up a plastic leaf]. LeaFF, do you hear our special sound?
>
> CHILD [vigorously shaking head]: Noooooo.

This is a listening game. Note that the child is not asked to say anything, just to listen for the TH in words. The clinician wants to be sure the child hears the sound before trying to teach how to say it. If there is homework after this lesson it may be for you to say some words which have the TH sound (a list should be provided by the clinician) and some which do not have it, and have your child tell you whether or not the TH sound is there. You will not ask your child to say the word; the yes and no answers are enough. If, however, your child does attempt to say the word, praise the right pronunciation but pass over the wrong pronunciation. At this point the wrong pronunciation is to be expected and the right pronunciation is a bonus.[13]

Another activity you might observe in the clinic if your child

13. C. Van Riper, *Speech Correction: Principles and Methods* (Englewood Cliffs, NJ: Prentice-Hall, 1978), Ch. 6. Van Riper describes "traditional therapy," which starts with ear training or listening training before any attempt to teach the child how to produce the problem sound. This is the most widespread method and is often called the Van Riper method (although not by Van Riper). It has worked successfully for years.

omits the final consonant of words is the following: A game is being played in which the child is forced to say the final consonant.

The clinician places five cards with pictures of bows on the table. Then five pictures of boats are spread on the table. Note, if you leave off the final sound of *boat* it becomes *bow*.

> CLINICIAN: Show me a picture of a bow. [Child points to bow.]
> CLINICIAN: Show me a picture of a boat. [Child points to a boat.]

This procedure is repeated a few times in order for the clinician to make sure the child can hear the difference between *bow* and *boat*.

> CLINICIAN: Let's play a game. You tell me what you want. I'll give you just what you say. If I give you a boat, you get a point. OK, what do you want?
> CHILD: I want a bow.
> CLINICIAN [handing child a bow]: Here it is.
> CHILD: No, I want a *bow!*
> CLINICIAN: OK [handing a bow]. I thought you would want a boaT.
> CHILD: Yeah, give me a bow . . . TT!
> CLINICIAN [handing over a boat]: One point for you.[14]

After this lesson the parent can reinforce it by picking out words ending in T and practicing them together, such as streeT, caT, lighT and so forth.

As you can see from these clinic dialogues, there is nothing particularly magic about speech therapy. The learning process is about the same whether it takes place without any direction or in the clinic or in school. The only thing the speech clinician really does is to break down the learning task into small bits. Some children need this. For instance your child will have to learn to listen to the trouble sound by itself and tell the difference between that sound and all the other sounds. Then your child will have to learn to differentiate that sound from the others when it is used in sylla-

---

14. F. Weiner, "Meaningful Minimal Contrast," *Journal of Speech and Hearing Disorders*, vol. 46, no. 1, 1981. This method is described. It is one of the relatively new programs and plans for treatment of articulation disorders in children. It is based on the idea that there are certain ways that children's speech deviates from that of adults. There is a system of mistakes rather than simply a collection of erred sounds. This method forces the child to use the adult speech pattern. Other child deviations are: cluster reduction (*boo* for *blue*, *fas* for *fast*), making hard contact sounds in place of soft contact sounds (*pish* for *fish*, *tun* for *sun*.) I think this method is a good one to incorporate the already learned sounds into new words.

bles or nonsense words. From there your child will have to move on to hearing the trouble sound in real words and judging whether the clinician pronounces it correctly or not. All this before your child is asked to pronounce a single thing. The actual pronunciation learning is broken down into small steps: single sound, syllables, words and sentences. Most of these activities can be repeated at home and are often assigned for extra practice.

What You Can Do

All the children we have seen have unclear speech without easily explained causes except for Nancy, who has other difficulties overlaid on her word-forming problems and may also have some kind of nerve or brain damage. They do not have anything wrong with their hearing, they are not brain damaged, they have no physical deformities, they are not unintelligent. In fact, other than the way they talk, they seem a pretty normal bunch. Some of their personal idiosyncrasies are probably due to their difficulty in speaking. Although we can make some guesses on what might have been the cause of the problem with each of these children, no one can state definitely what is the cause and what is not. There may be one or a combination of causes. And even knowing the cause does not automatically tell the parents what to do about it.

Provide a good adult speech model. Whether or not you think your child has a speech problem, give the youngster as much chance as possible to hear speech spoken correctly. It does not have to be complicated formal speech with complex sentences and big words, but rather it should be simple, clear and correct. Parents should avoid using baby talk themselves. If a baby hears "Look at the witto babykins go beddy bye" as a model for the kind of talk to learn, don't be surprised if the baby grows into childhood talking like that.

Expect better pronunciation as your child grows older. Become fussy little by little. If your two-year-old says *muk* for *milk*, accept that for the time being. But don't *you* slip into calling it *muk*. Always use the work *milk* and emphasize the L as *millllllk*. Make sure the baby has plenty of time to hear the word said right. At two and a half or three you might decide you've had enough of *muk* and that the child ought to improve pronunciation. Now you say "What do you want?" when the child says *muk*. Don't tell your child that *muk* is wrong and that the word must be said *milk*. Just pretend not to understand a couple of times until you see the child making an effort with the word. When the child tries to refine the pronunciation of the word somewhat, even if the result is not perfect, you can suddenly understand and say, "Oh, you mean milllllk." Be aware that words go through all sorts of stages while being perfected. Thus *muk* can change to *mook* then to *mil* and finally arrive at *milk*. As long as the mispronounced word is changing in its sound you need not worry. If your baby or child said a word one way last week and says it differently this week (and both are wrong), that word and the sounds in that word have not yet settled down. The child is still in the process of learning, and your role in that process is to be there with the correct pronunciation so that the child can always have a standard to work toward and to compare to. Don't demand perfection in order to understand too soon; that leads to discouragement and frustration. You can also help your child by playing imitation games: do-what-I-do and say-what-I-say games. The results don't have to be judged, just playing them is enough. Singing songs is also effective. Often the rhythm helps the child imitate the grownup word. Be patient, don't expect perfection, but do expect progress.

Provide extra stimulation for trouble sounds you hear. When you feel your child has developed some habits of mistaken pronunciation, make a list of the mispronounced words for yourself without your child being aware of it. Remember one of those mispronounced words and try to load your conversation with it for one day. Don't expect your child to say it back, just hearing it many times during the day is important. The next day do the same thing with another one of the words on your list. Go through about six words in six days then start the cycle all over again. These should be natural words for you to use every day as you got them from your child. Continue for about a month and listen critically to these words again. Judge whether or not there is any change in pronunciation. Your child may be able to learn the natural way with just a little extra stimulation from you. What you will be providing will be better than speech therapy.

What to Expect from Your Child's Speech

At a year old, your baby will be attempting a few words. You will probably not be able to understand them immediately. There are probably many parents who miss their baby's first words because they don't sound like words. There are also parents who think they heard their baby say words that were actually never said. As your baby uses more and more words you will become increasingly better able to understand them. You should be aware of the meaning of some of your child's speech but not necessarily all of it by the age of two or two and a half; however, don't expect anyone else to understand it. By three your child should be understood by sympathetic and attentive listeners outside the immediate family. By four years everyone should be able to understand your child's speech even though there may still be words that are not pronounced right. By the time your child is ready to go to first grade all the sounds should be pronounced correctly although there may be some trouble with certain sound combinations.

How You Can Help Your Child at Home Without Speech Therapy

It is not necessary to wait for speech therapy if you want to help your child pronounce words clearly. Without replacing the speech pathologist, you can adopt some general principles to help your child. First, speech learning should be a fun-filled, anxiety-free, positive activity. Your child should never feel "put on the spot" to pronounce perfectly. You should be tolerant of the many trip-ups and mistakes that are part of the learning process. It is often hard for your child to understand that your disapproval of poor speech is not disapproval of the child as a person. Speech is such a very personal expression that it is difficult for any of us to separate disapproval of how we are talking from what we are saying. And it is hard to separate disapproval of what we are saying from disapproval of ourselves. Your child needs assurance of your love, admiration and approval no matter how many mistakes you hear.

Second, you should be sure your own speech is slow and clear enough for your child to hear all the sounds. If a whole word is too big a mouthful, try part of a word or even a single sound if you can find it. Read books and stories to your child. The alphabet books are good, not so much to teach the letters but because they feature certain sounds in a clear way such as B is for *ball*. Both you and your child can see how a sound fits into words. Make certain that these books use a letter that really does represent the sound. K is for *king* is fine, but K is for *knife* is confusing. The G for *girl* is different from the G for *giraffe*. Remember that letters have different names from the sounds they represent. The letter B (bee) doesn't go into *ball* by its name. The "B" part stands for what you do with your lips before you continue with the *all* part of *ball*.

Patience is probably the most important quality you need to help your child with pronunciation. Children don't acquire clear speech overnight under the best of circumstances. If your child needs extra help, the learning process can seem agonizingly slow. Remember it takes time to learn a high-speed high-precision skill such as talking perfectly.

Suggestions for Parents of Children with Unclear Speech

- Understand that for many normal children it takes until school age for all the sounds to be learned.
- Don't correct your child in a negative manner.
- Provide your child with the correct model of the mispronounced word, emphasizing and prolonging the trouble sound.
- Don't be *too* understanding. If you think your child can say a word better, fail to understand until you notice an effort at improvement.
- On the other hand do not demand perfection of pronunciation when such an expectation is unrealistic.
- Encourage speech sound games and rhymes such as "Fee fie fo fum" etc. even for sounds your child is not having trouble with.
- If your child's speech deteriorates, look for some emotional problem.
- Give your child experience in talking with unfamiliar people, people unused to your child's speaking style.
- Ask friends or relatives who do not hear your child's speech every day if they notice changes in your child's speech skill.
- Be alert that pronunciation may not be your child's only speech problem. There could be language formation problems as well.
- Do not ridicule or allow others (if you can help it) to ridicule your child's speech.
- Do not expect your child to "grow out" of unclear speech after seven years of age. Seek help.
- If your child is receiving treatment, reinforce at home with a clinician's advice.

6

How to Help Your Child with a Cleft Lip or Cleft Palate

The joy Martha's parents felt at the successful birth of a daughter turned to shock and dismay when they first saw their infant's face. There was a crooked hole in the place where her mouth should have been. Her lip was twisted up toward her nose. An oral surgeon explained Martha's condition to her parents. Martha was born with a cleft lip and palate, but, even though Martha looked hopelessly deformed right now, with proper treatment she would grow up without noticeable disfigurement or speech problems.

Martha's first few weeks of life presented many difficulties for her parents. They experimented with several methods of feeding because Martha's lip and mouth deformity made it impossible for her to suck normally. There was also no way for Martha to close off her nose from her mouth so that the food that did get in her mouth tended to run out her nose. Many of these feeding problems would be fixed by surgery, but Martha would have to weigh at least ten pounds before such surgery could be performed.

What Is Cleft Palate or Lip?

Oral clefts are a congenital deformity. The upper jaw and the front portion of the nose (all making up the maxilla) start out as three separate structures in the embryo. The forward part includes the front part of the nose and the upper jaw with the four front teeth. There are two back parts which become either side of the hard palate (the bony part of the roof of the mouth) and either side of the soft palate just in back of the hard palate. These structures join or fuse at different stages of embryonic development into the single rigid structure that most people have.[1] In medieval times cleft lip was called hare lip because the divided lip looked like the lip formation of a rabbit or hare. It was thought that hare lip was caused by a woman looking at a hare while pregnant. Nowadays we think that some cases can be caused by hereditary factors.[2] In other cases it can be caused by injury or by drugs taken by the pregnant mother which interfere with normal embryonic development so that the three palate parts fail to come together or fail to come together completely. It is also possible that the condition is caused by certain infections suffered by the pregnant mother at critical stages in the child's prenatal life. But in many instances it is impossible to determine the cause, and there is still much to be learned about why facial clefts occur. We do know that oral clefts are more common in some parts of the world than others and that they vary widely among different races. They occur once in about every 750 live births among whites, once in 400 live births among Asians and once in about 2500 births among blacks. They are also more frequent among American Indians than other Americans.

Facial clefts can vary in type and degree. The clefts at the front can be on either one side or the other or both and involve the lip, the gum, the front part of the hard palate or any combination

1. G. Powers, *Cleft Palate* (Indianapolis: Bobbs-Merrill Educational Publishing, 1973). It is thought that cleft lips are due to a fusing failure approximately six weeks after conception. Cleft palate is a failure occurring in the ninth week of embryonic life.

2. While the role heredity plays in the cause of facial clefts is not clear, the cleft lip seems to have a greater heredity factor than the cleft palate or cleft of both lip and palate.

There have been animal studies (Powers, 1973) in which pregnant animals were given drugs or toxins or radiation or diets with certain deficiencies, whose offspring showed a greater prevalence than normal of facial clefts. It is not clear how these findings relate to causes of facial clefts in humans.

of these structures. They can be wide or small. Clefts farther back in the mouth are down the middle and can be in the hard palate, the soft palate or both. The least severe deformity of this kind is a bifid uvula in which the little piece of flesh which hangs down at the back of the mouth is divided in two so that it looks like two uvulas. Cleft lips are the most disfiguring, but the palatal clefts may be more serious, often being combined with other problems. One such problem may be that the muscles necessary to close off the mouth from the nose may be affected and not function properly even after the bony part of the palate is repaired surgically.

Problems of Facial Cleft Children

The earliest problem encountered by parents, after first getting used to the deformity, is feeding. Because each different individual presents a different feeding difficulty there are a variety of approaches. Sometimes surgery is done very early in the baby's life. Sometimes a modified nursing nipple or syringe is effective. An obdurator, a device made of plastic to be fitted over the roof of the mouth similar to the retainer worn by people having their teeth straightened by an orthodontist, solved the feeding dilemma for Martha's parents.

The next worry the parents have is that the hearing of the oral cleft child is in jeopardy. Sometimes the deformity also affects the ear structure enough to impair hearing. Danger arises because during eating there is bound to be some drainage of milk through the nose which can then drain into the baby's ears. Martha's parents found that Martha was sensitive about her ears in the first few months. If someone touched her near her ear she reacted as if she were in pain. Sometimes she did not notice sounds in her environment. Probably Martha's ears were often stopped up, impairing her hearing. Of course, even without an earache any chronic congestion in a baby's ears is cause for concern. Martha's pediatrician explained that the danger was that the temporary hearing loss brought on by congestion could become a permanent hearing loss and that Martha's speech and language development could be threatened. Moreover, this condition predisposes a child to ear infections. Before the widespread use of antibiotics to treat infection, many children with facial clefts grew up unable to speak properly, not because the physical deformity prevented them from forming words but because hearing loss impaired their language. The doctor assured Martha's parents that such damage to Martha's hearing could be prevented if they were careful to watch the baby and take action at the first sign of ear trouble.

Speech Progress in a Facial Cleft Child

Martha was six months old when she had her first operation. The surgeon closed her lip. The cosmetic results were startling. Her face became beautiful; there was no longer a hole where there should have been an upper lip. The oral surgeon and the plastic surgeon were concerned not only with her ability to eat but with her looks. For the first time Martha's parents believed that their daughter's face would not be deformed for the rest of her life. The cleft palate team at the hospital cautioned the parents that there would be other operations. The scar left from the first operation could be reduced and maybe eliminated completely in time, but there would be another operation when Martha would be a year old to close up the bony part of the cleft. Further operations might be needed to place the teeth when they came in and to help Martha close off her nose from her mouth.

Martha said her first word at two years. This is later than usual, but her parents did not expect her to follow a normal timetable because her situation was not normal. The operations and frequent earaches would have slowed her down even without the cleft.

Like many parents of handicapped children, Martha's parents did not compare her progress to that of normal children, but welcomed each developmental milestone whenever it came. Soon the words came tumbling out. They had expected that Martha's voice would have the nasal quality common to many cleft palate people, so they were pleasantly surprised when her voice turned out to be normal for a girl of her age. Martha's words were pronounced as clearly as any two-and-a-half-year-old's. The pediatrician still recommended that Martha have speech therapy. Her parents were surprised because they felt that it really did not seem necessary for Martha. Martha did substitute some sounds for others, but didn't all children her age do that?

Nevertheless, because the pediatrician thought that Martha should be checked, her parents took her to a speech/language pathologist. They discovered that Martha did have a normal number of speech mistakes—but not the normal *kind* of mistakes. Martha said *kish* instead of *fish* and *gig* instead of *big*. Usually children master sounds made with the front part of the mouth and the lips (F and B) before they master sounds made with the back part of the mouth (K and hard G). Her cleft had been in the front part of the mouth, and her mistakes in speech seemed an attempt to avoid using that part. Perhaps Martha had missed out on the P's and B's and F's in the babbling stage of her babyhood and needed help in finding and using these structures now that they were repaired. The speech clinician further explained that there were some sounds that Martha was producing normally now that could deteriorate as she grew older. As Martha grows older her head will lengthen and the gap between her soft palate and her throat (which is normally closed off by lifting the soft palate until it touches the back of the throat during speaking) will grow larger. This means that Martha will have a more difficult task closing off her nose from her mouth (velopharyngeal closure). Moreover her adenoids are a little bit enlarged now and help in blocking off the back of her nose, they will shrink in time.

All the sounds except M, N and NG are made through the mouth. Some speech sounds need a fair amount of breath pressure in the mouth and cannot be produced if some of the air escapes out the nose. If Martha starts speech therapy early, while her velopharyngeal mechanism is working easily, she can conserve the good speech quality she has. It is easier to keep good speaking habits than to let the speech deteriorate and try to get them back. By playing sound games in the clinic and continuing them at home it is hoped that Martha's muscles will be strengthened so that when the time comes in which the closure is more difficult, she will be able to make the extra necessary effort.

When Martha and her mother took walks together, they could be heard practicing *pah pah pah* in time with each step. They did blowing exercises together. Martha's mother would hold a lighted candle and Martha would be asked to make the flame dance by blowing. The idea of the exercise is for Martha to direct the breath from her mouth on the candle flame. If the velopharyngeal valve were not closed adequately the breath stream would escape out the nose, not leaving enough breath in the mouth to make the flame dance. As Martha concentrates on the flame she would make the right kind of effort to close off her nose.

While these exercises are fun for Martha and her parents, Martha's velopharyngeal valve would get better exercise for its speaking needs by using speaking. An example of such an exercise would be to say sibilant syllables such as *ssssay sssso sssaw*. The air has to be held in the mouth to say these syllables correctly. Syllables with P, K, T (*pah* or *eep, koo, ahk, tay, oot* or using any other vowels) require a lot of breath pressure to pronounce clearly and would make better syllables to exercise velopharyngeal closure than the syllables using G, B and D. Syllables or words with S, F, TH (as in *thin*) and SH require a sustained breath pressure and can be used with children like Martha. Martha's mother was not teaching her speaking motions that she did not already know but practicing and reinforcing sounds already learned. Most children like sound games and rhyming and nonsense words, and Martha thought that she was playing.

Martha had speech therapy for a few months when she was three and a half. Her parents continued doing the activities the speech clinician suggested and reevaluated her speech every six months until she went to school. When Martha did go to school her speech was normal. The school speech clinician in the school speech screening program was the only one to notice the faint scar on the side of Martha's upper lip. Martha's speech, however, had nothing in it to suggest even to the trained listener that there had been anything wrong with her.

Not every child like Martha turns out so well. It would be hard to say which factor was the crucial one. She was a lucky child to be cared for by a cleft palate team of several professionals: an oral surgeon, an orthodontist, a plastic surgeon, a pediatrician, an audiologist and a speech language pathologist. But most important she was lucky to have parents who were creative, resourceful and caring.

Helping the Child Whose Speech Problems Do Not Clear up Before Entering School

Ellen at ten years old does not look too different from other children her age. If you look at her closely, however, you will notice two small scars on either side of her upper lip. When Ellen was born her face was more deformed than Martha's. She had an opening on both sides of her lip. In her short life Ellen has had eleven operations to repair the cleft lip and also to repair the clefts on either side of her upper jaw. All the surgery has paid off. Her face looks normal. Her upper lip is a bit shorter than it might be, but not in any way one might think abnormal. Many people have naturally short upper lips.

The first year of Ellen's life was very difficult for her parents. They were ashamed of their baby's looks and they would not take her out where other people would see her. They never adequately solved the many feeding problems they had with her. She did not gain weight at a reassuring rate nor did she seem robust. She had recurring earaches with fever which worried her parents. At four months Ellen had her first operation, which relieved the feeding problems somewhat. The earaches continued to be a regular part of her life. Very often the operations which followed had to be rescheduled many times because of the recurring ear infections.

Ellen attempted to say her first word when she was nearly three years old. Earlier when she tried babbling one or the other parent would pick her up and attempt to distract her from making the vocalizations. When she started trying to talk her parents tried to stop her. They had two reasons: one was to let the most recent operation heal properly, and the other was that they thought it would be bad for her to try to talk until her mouth was "finished" as she might talk wrong and learn bad habits. They did not realize that Ellen was in her best years for learning how to speak. They also did not realize that with the recurring infections in her ears, her perception of other people's speech was often muffled. Nobody listened closely enough to the little amount of talking she did to notice the mistakes in her speech. During the preschool years, as she grew older and more robust, her ears cleared up. Aside from frequent hospital stays for an operation on her mouth she was a pretty healthy little girl. In first grade she went to a church-affiliated school that did not have speech therapy services. In spite of her poor start in life she did fine in her academic subjects: reading, writing, math, language arts. When she had to read aloud, however, the other children teased her because she sounded funny. The teacher, trying to be tactful, stopped calling on her to read aloud. On the playground she suffered the stigma of being different.

How was her speech different? Her S and Z sounds sounded like snorts. Her SH and F and V sounds were muffled. Ellen was aware of the snorting and tried to prevent it. Since she could not hold back the air from her nose by moving her soft palate, she twitched her nostrils instead. Not only did she sound funny, she also looked funny. At home when she talked and constricted her nostrils she was reprimanded. Her parents thought it was simply an annoying habit she had picked up, not understanding that it was Ellen's attempt at making her speech more acceptable. Unfortunately, holding the nose will not help eliminate nasal resonance although it will stop the escape of air through the nostrils. Ellen's mother did notice something about her daughter's speech that she thought might be related to the oral cleft. Sometimes when Ellen said a word like *bottle* or *apple* there would be a funny noise like a click in the throat instead of the middle consonant. Ellen's mother was quite right in thinking it was related to the cleft. Ellen had avoided the more forward parts of her mouth (where the P and T are normally produced) and tried to approximate these sounds with the back of the throat. This sound is called a glottal catch. It not only sounds peculiar but if you do it too much it hurts. Ellen did indeed sound funny. She had snorted S's, muffled sounds and glottal catches which gave her speech a jerky sound. Added to all this was the nasal twitching.

When Ellen was in the fourth grade the family moved to a different town. Speech and language services were available in the new school as part of the school program. So for the first time Ellen had speech therapy. The school clinician admired the beautiful job the surgeons had done in restructuring Ellen's mouth. There was no reason Ellen could not speak normally as far as the physical makeup of her mouth was concerned. The speech clinician conferred with Ellen's parents and worked out a program at school and at home to help Ellen's speech.

Ellen was so conscious of her nose and how much it was contributing to her problem that she was concentrating her efforts on stopping her nose. She told the speech clinician that she knew she talked through her nose but did not know how to stop it. To make Ellen more mouth conscious, to teach her to "think mouth," the speech teacher painted her mouth with bright red lipstick, then told her to say some words as she looked at herself in the mirror. Of course the visual impression she got from her image was all mouth and her nose was hardly seen. The clinician wanted to give her a more vivid image of how words come out of the mouth. She pulled an imaginary string, representing words, from Ellen's mouth as she was talking. During several conferences with Ellen's parents, the clinician convinced them that speaking was not going to harm Ellen's mouth and that the only way she could learn to talk well would be to practice her speech at home. For home practice sessions both Ellen and her mother made up their mouths with bright red lipstick and both looked into the mirror as they talked together. Interestingly, Ellen's mother did not see the nasal twitches when her daughter's mouth was painted up. Perhaps her eye and therefore her attention was drawn to Ellen's mouth. Or perhaps with Ellen more conscious of her mouth she did not try so hard to constrict her nose. Mother and daughter had fun painting themselves up in different styles (always emphasizing the mouth), and for the first time Ellen's mother enjoyed helping her child. Ellen's father became used to finding the ladies of the house made up like clowns when he came home from work.

Ellen and her parents thought that the glottal catches were the most distressing part of Ellen's speech. They tried an exercise the speech clinician suggested. The parent would give Ellen a syllable to say twice, such as *pa*. The first *pa* was while Ellen was sucking in air and the second *pa* on breathing out. They would do this several times in unison. Both Ellen and her parent had to be careful at first so that they would not hyperventilate and become dizzy. It is impossible or at least very hard to do a glottal catch while breathing in. Ellen was forced to use her lips to form the P in *pa* on the inhalation because she couldn't do her customary glottal catch. She maintained the correct lip production for the P on the second syllable which was made with exhaled breath as is all normal speech. They worked with syllables with other consonant sounds: B, T, K, D and hard G. The second exercise was to do the same thing using words such as *boy* or *do*. *Boy* (sucking in) *boy* (breathing out). *Do* (sucking in) *do* (breathing out). The third exercise of this series used the same words Ellen had trouble with, like *pickle* and *battle*. This time they exhaled on the first syllable and inhaled on the second. *Ba* (breathing out) *ttle* (sucking in). *Pi* (breathing out) *ckle* (sucking in). These exercises led Ellen into the correct pronunciation, the drill got her used to the feel of the correct production, and she became able to say these words correctly without the inhaled speech.

At school Ellen learned to evaluate nasality in other people's speech. Her own speech was recorded and she was asked to evaluate the nasal quality of her own speech as she listened to it play back. Strangely she was less able to evaluate the nasality of her own speech than she was for other people's speech. Perhaps she was too emotionally involved listening to her own speech to make objective judgments. The clinician guided her to hear the nasality in her own speech with some degree of accuracy. Another remedy for nasal speech involved encouraging Ellen to keep her mouth more open as she talked. She came to realize that the vowel sounds she made with a small mouth opening like the OO and the EE are more nasal-sounding than those made with a large mouth opening like the AH or the A in *hat*. What worked for the vowels worked for all speech. In order to help Ellen learn to talk with a more open mouth, she was instructed to put the tip of her thumb between the upper and lower front teeth, taking care not to bite down too hard and try to talk as normally as possible. If you try this yourself you will find that it takes more effort to talk clearly but you can speak pretty well. After Ellen had talked through her thumb a few minutes her pronunciation was clearer and more precise when she took away her thumb. This exercise can also be done with a small plastic wedge between the teeth which makes it easier to say the lip sounds like P and B. (Parents of young children should be careful of using any device for speech which could be swallowed by the child.) Thus Ellen learned how to talk with her mouth more open and still talk clearly.

Another exercise for helping Ellen control her nasal resonance was saying syllables rapidly (such as *pa pa pa*) while holding a small mirror under her nose and looking into a large mirror. If the small mirror does not fog, she is saying it correctly without an escape of air through her nose. If she sees the mirror cloud up, she is breathing out through her nose. She can practice at home watching the mirror to make sure it doesn't fog. Of course if the syllables include M, N or NG the mirror should fog. If she stops talking, the mirror will also fog because we naturally breathe out through our nose when we are not talking. The speech teacher thought that this exercise would help Ellen control her velopharyngeal valve better than the traditional blowing exercises. The rapid opening and closing of the valve used in speaking is different from the tighter and more static closing of the valve necessary for blowing up balloons.[3] Some nasal emission of air is normal in talking. Try doing Ellen's exercise while carrying on a normal conversation and you will see that your mirror will be fogged to some extent. In fact totally non-nasal speech does not sound too good. But as an exercise for a child like Ellen it was effective.

Ellen's speech seemed to improve when she learned to lower the pitch of her voice. For some reason a high voice sounds more nasal. She practiced this low voice on her portable tape recorder at home. The resulting voice was not abnormally low for a girl of her age, just at the low end of her normal range. As she grows older her voice pitch will naturally drop. Ellen's parents gave her a small cassette tape recorder and found that she was able to use it to practice her speech by herself. She gained a more realistic idea of what her tape recorded voice sounded like.

An unexpected outcome of Ellen's speech therapy and improvement in talking was that her appearance changed for the better. Before the therapy both Ellen and her mother were conscious of the little scars on Ellen's upper lip. Most people would not have noticed them unless they were pointed out, but to Ellen's mother they were huge. She remembered when Ellen's face was really deformed and could not seem to get that image of her child out of her mind. She conveyed her attitude to Ellen without words, as such attitudes are often conveyed to children. Ellen felt she was ugly. She saw those little white lines as disfiguring. She took no interest in clothes, as do many ten-year-old girls, thinking that it did not matter what she wore because she would still be ugly. As Ellen's speech improved, her self-image improved. When she looked into the mirror (there was a lot of mirror work in her therapy) she had to admit what she saw was a pretty girl and even her mother came to see her that way. Ellen's mother, a beauty herself, had been bitterly disappointed that her child's face was deformed. But as she saw the effects of her daughter's poise and self-confidence the beauty she had always wanted began to emerge. Speech therapy won't always make a child beautiful, but

3. C. Van Riper, *Speech Correction: Principles and Practice* (Englewood Cliffs, NJ: Prentice-Hall, 1978). There are other therapeutic exercises for cleft palate children. A skilled speech pathologist can massage the area around the uvula lightly to strengthen the child's awareness of the palate. Closed-mouth yawning also helps the child become aware of palatal movement.

it can help others to see the beauty that was always there by making it possible for the child to come out of a shell of noncommunication and blossom as a result of increased clarity of speech, vitality and self-acceptance.

A Hidden Cleft Palate

Greg at ten has been in school speech therapy since the first grade. His speech is not so hard to understand, it just doesn't sound right. He has learned to produce all the sounds correctly, and when he says a single word he sounds fine. But when he speaks a longer speech segment, his sounds seem a little blurred and there is an unpleasant quality to his voice. One speech teacher remarked that Greg sounds as if he had a cleft palate. When his mouth was examined, however, it looked perfectly normal. The new speech teacher at school wanted to make sure and reexamined his mouth. The new teacher noticed that Greg's uvula was somewhat off center, which was odd, but that did not really indicate anything. But when Greg was asked to go *Ahh* while the clinician looked at his soft palate to see how it moved, it didn't snap up the way other children's soft palates do; the movement was sluggish. This was not surprising because Greg's speech quality suggested that his soft palate was not moving too well. The clinician also noticed a faintly bluish color on the roof of his mouth, which is normally pinkish. The difference in color was so subtle that it could easily have been missed. Still wanting to know why Greg's soft palate was not moving well, the teacher pressed the top part of the roof of his mouth with a tongue blade as gently as possible. Some of the parts which should have been bony and hard seemed soft. An X-ray picture of Greg's palate would have given a better view but the speech clinician did not have access to an X-ray machine. Nonetheless, it was decided his speech problem should be viewed in a different way. Greg's pronunciation problem was thought to be a result of poor learning of speech sounds, a common speech difficulty in schoolchildren. The speech teacher thought, however, that the real reason for Greg's poor speech was that he had a cleft palate which was invisible because it was covered over by the fleshy skin of the roof of his mouth. The cleft was probably a series of holes or perforations in the bone along the fusion line. He did not have the many other problems cleft palate children have in babyhood, nor did he suffer the deformity Martha had. No one had worried about

Greg's speech. Everyone assumed he was normal. Although the palate was closed over by soft flesh, the muscles of the palate and the throat did not work as well as they had to in order to close off Greg's nose.[4] In normal people this velopharyngeal mechanism makes such a closing very easy. It is "overengineered," meaning that there is more ability than is absolutely necessary. But Greg could close off his nose only sometimes and only with effort because his velopharyngeal mechanism worked partially at best. If his parents had known about the problem early enough they might have had some speech help for him so that he could maintain the velopharyngeal closure he had had when he was little. But since the problem was invisible it was (not surprisingly) overlooked. The speech teacher decided to help Greg work around his sluggish closure mechanism. Speech therapy in the past had aggravated the voice quality in Greg's speech. The new speech teacher taught Greg to form his consonant sounds with as soft and as loose a contact as possible. This is almost the opposite of most speech therapy, which encourages sharp precise pronunciation. Greg was also encouraged to talk with his mouth as open as possible. At first he objected to this, as it made him feel silly. But he tried it and it seemed to work. The idea behind this is that if the mouth is wide open the air will more likely flow through this large opening than through the smaller opening of the nose. The hard tight contact that Greg had been taught earlier to make his consonant sound clear tended to reduce his mouth size and build up more pressure than necessary. It forced the air out through every available route including the nose, giving his speech a snorting sound that was distinctly unpleasant. In order to compensate for the soft loose speaking style, Greg was encouraged to prolong his speech sounds, making them easier to understand.

Greg's parents had become used to Greg's speech and had long since given up hope that it could be improved. They were delighted and surprised to hear the improvement at home as he tried out his new speech. Greg's mother made an appointment with the speech teacher to say how pleased she was. The clinician explained the theory behind the new treatment of Greg's speech. At first

4. S. Ewanowski and J. H. Saxman, "Orafacial Disorders" from *Introduction to Communication Disorders*, ed. by T. J. Hixon, L. D. Shriberg and T. J. Saxman (Englewood Cliffs, NJ: Prentice-Hall, 1980). A careful examination could have been made by an expert by feeling the central part of the palate with a rubber finger or covering. If Greg had had a bifid uvula the condition would have been more obvious.

Greg's mother was shocked, not being able to believe that Greg could have had a deformity at birth. She asked whether she should take Greg to a doctor to have his mouth X-rayed. As they talked, however, his mother decided that there was no need to have the X-rays, because the speech and voice problems Greg had had from the invisible (or submucous) cleft were in the process of being fixed. The speech teacher further explained that even if Greg were to have surgery he would still need speech therapy to learn to use the new physical structure. The speech teacher and the mother decided to see if speech therapy alone could do the job for Greg. As it turned out he developed acceptable speech both in pronunciation and in quality by learning this new pattern of speaking. Sometimes speech pathologists have to teach an alternative method of speaking to compensate for an imperfect speech mechanism instead of teaching the customary speech patterns.

If speech therapy had not been enough to help Greg overcome his nasal tone of voice, he could have undergone a surgical treatment called the pharyngeal flap. In this operation a flap of skin taken from the back of the throat is used as a bridge over the pharyngeal opening, thus creating normal functioning of the palate throat mechanism. This operation is often performed on people with cleft palates as part of the constructive surgical remediation. It is also done for people without a history of oral cleft who have persistent nasal resonance voice problems. When the imperfect structure makes closing off the nose from the mouth impossible for a child, no amount of speech therapy will correct the nasality in the voice and therefore surgery is necessary.[5] In Greg's case there was some structural inadequacy but not enough to make such closure really impossible. Therefore the nonsurgical or braining approach seemed most appropriate.

Good Treatment Can Reduce the Handicap of Facial Clefts

Cleft palate and/or lip is a birth defect which is probably at its worst in the beginning. Proper treatment can make the deformity and the speech difficulty seem not as bad as they did at first. Surgery to restore and construct mouth functioning has improved greatly in the last few years.

5. Another surgical or really prosthetic technique is the Teflon implant in the pharynx. The mass of Teflon makes the back of the throat bulge forward, making it easier for the short and not so mobile soft palate to close the gap.

Parents are often particularly distressed when a daughter has a cleft lip; not only will her looks be affected, but she won't be able to hide her scar with a mustache when she grows up. Today's modern plastic surgery is so skillful, however, that there is often nothing left to hide.[6] Oral surgery, prosthodontics (the fitting of appliances to aid functioning) and orthodontics can give the facial cleft child good-looking, well-functioning oral structures. Speech therapy should be included in this team effort. But the parents are the most important part of this team. Old attitudes about birth defects in general and "hare lip" in particular must be overcome. It takes time, patience and money to do the complete repair job, and it is not without considerable pain and discomfort for your child. Moreover, there is considerable work for your child on speech, both to prevent speech problems and to remedy speech problems already developed. This requires parents to exercise even more care and patience. But the results are worth it. Remember that although facial clefts are not common, they are not as rare as you might think. You have passed many people born with this condition and have not been aware of it. Strangers passing your child will also not be aware of the deformity that once caused such worry.

Suggestions for Parents of Children with Facial Clefts

- Be prepared for several operations to repair the cleft.
- Try to have your child treated by a team of different professionals: oral surgeon, prosthodontist, speech pathologist, audiologist, psychologist, to name a few members of the team.
- Be sure to offer your child more than the usual language-building stimulation.
- Encourage babbling, vocal play and speech as much as possible.
- Be alert for hearing problems.
- Even if your child's speech seems all right in the years just before school, consult a speech pathologist to avoid problems later on.
- If your older child with a repaired cleft still has poor voice quality, consult a speech pathologist. Nasality can be helped.
- Even if surgery or prosthesis restores your child's speech structure, enabling perfect speech production, it still takes time for your child to learn to use the new structure.

6. Girls with facial clefts have an advantage over boys because they have available, from the genital area, more of the type of skin suitable for skin grafts inside the mouth.

7

How to Help Your Cerebral Palsied Child

- *What Is Cerebral Palsy?*
- *Help for the Cerebral Palsied Child*
- *The Nontalker*
- *The Clumsy Child: A Mild Case of Cerebral Palsy*
- *Cerebral Palsy Covers a Wide Range of Handicapping Conditions*
- *Suggestions for the Parents of Children with Cerebral Palsy*

Luis was born prematurely. After a difficult birth and a tense two weeks of fears for his survival, he seemed to settle down and thrive like any normal baby. There was some difficulty getting him to nurse, but his parents thought this was because of his prematurity. Each parent had private fears, however, that Luis would suffer aftereffects from his two-week bout with breathing problems. By the time Luis was six months old, the time that normal babies begin to sit up by themselves, he was not able to hold up his head or to roll over. Luis's parents noticed that he would tense all his muscles at once every time he moved at all. At nine months, when other babies are beginning to crawl around, Luis finally mastered holding up his head. His parents realized that his development was late; the experience of those frightening first two weeks had prepared them for the possibility. Although they had shared their concern with their son's pediatrician, it was not until Luis was one year old that the doctor made a definite diagnosis: he told them that their son had cerebral palsy. They asked him what it meant to have cerebral palsy. The only time they had heard the term was on a television program on various birth defects which had shown a severely crippled child who was a victim of cerebral palsy. Luis's parents were devastated to imagine that their son would always be a hopeless cripple. The doctor tried to explain that cerebral palsy did not always mean severe crippling and in fact the term covered many different conditions.

What Is Cerebral Palsy?

The term "cerebral palsy" is used to include a wide range of disabilities of the motor system (ability to move) brought on by damage to the brain. Most say this damage occurs either before birth, during delivery or shortly after birth. Sometimes the term is used to refer to motor problems acquired later as a result of accident or stroke. There are all degrees of severity, from a person who seems just on the clumsy side of normal to someone who is totally crippled (unable to care for basic needs). It can affect some parts or all of the body. There are also many different ways cerebral palsy can impair the motor system: there can be paralysis (inability to move), weakness, poor coordination, inability to relax muscles, and involuntary movements or tremors. The victim may be unable to hold an object or unable to let it go. The likelihood is that there will be more than one of these types of impairment.[1]

Causes of Cerebral Palsy

Cerebral palsy has probably always been with us. Ancient Egyptian sculptures show figures in postures typical of cerebral palsied persons. Before the beginnings of scientific medicine in the nineteenth century, cerebral palsy was rare. Babies who had suffered the types of conditions which resulted in this injury to the brain did not live. In the last century many of these babies were saved only to survive handicapped. In the last half of the twentieth century cerebral palsy has become less common and the cases which do occur are less severe. Medical techniques such as thor-

1. Cerebral palsied children are divided into groups according to symptoms: spastic, exaggerated stretching during attempts to move; athetoid, involuntary tremors and flailing during muscle activity; rigid, all the muscles contracts locking the body immobile; tremor, rhythmic contraction of muscles at rest while not trying to move or the other way around. One or more of these symptoms may be present in any given case. There are also accompanying problems: convulsions, mental retardation, emotional problems, perceptual problems, hyperactivity, hearing loss, poor vision.

ough prenatal care, fetal monitoring during labor and better premature infant care have advanced to the point that not only can the babies be saved but brain damage can often be avoided. (But not always, as Luis's parents realized.)

Some of the causes of cerebral palsy are German measles, chicken pox, mumps and other viral diseases during pregnancy, blood type incompatibility (Rh factor), diabetes and pregnancy problems such as toxemia. Deprivation of oxygen is the major cause of damage to the infant's brain just before, during or right after birth. An infant is particularly vulnerable when undergoing the rigors of labor and in the changeover from the placental oxygen supply system to lung breathing. Prior pregnancy problems make this time around birth an especially risky one. Another cause of cerebral palsy, trauma to the brain, does damage because it deprives the affected parts of oxygen.[2]

Estimates of the incidence of cerebral palsy vary from as high as nineteen per thousand live births to as low as three per thousand. One reason for the difference in prevalence estimates is the wide range of severity from the severely crippled to the barely impaired. There are probably many children with such a mild case of cerebral palsy, with so few outward signs, that doctors, parents and teachers may only suspect, or may not even be aware of, the condition. Such children would not be included in any survey.

Problems of the Cerebral Palsied Child

Luis's parents have seen that there is some motor development although it is slow. At one year he is rolling over on his own. But will he eventually catch up to other children? His parents have noticed that Luis's movements are different as well as being immature. He may have trouble not only in coordinating the movements necessary for walking but in keeping his balance. He may have problems in handling and manipulating things. The supposedly

2. Some experts believe that up to 40 percent of cerebral palsy is inherited. Aside from the viral diseases which directly damage the developing fetal brain, the most common prenatal acquired cause is lack of oxygen. Umbilical cord and placenta problems can be responsible. Anemia, carbon monoxide poisoning, and breathing problems from drugs are problems the pregnant mother can have. At birth the baby may have problems starting breathing. Babies delivered by Caesarian section are in greater danger of having cerebral palsy. After birth the danger to the baby are trauma and infection. It must be remembered, however, that many babies undergo these events without acquiring cerebral palsy.

simple dressing, grooming, toilet and feeding skills may be difficult for him to learn. At any rate Luis will be slower in learning them, keeping him dependent on the care of others longer than usual. He may have hearing, vision and perceptual problems: either poor eyesight or hearing loss or the inability to interpret what he hears and sees. There is a good possibility that Luis will also have speech problems because speech requires so much coordination and precise fine movements. It may be that he will not be able to coordinate his exhaling with activating his voice box. Or he may not be able to make the rapid tongue movements necessary for clear speech. Control of his jaws and his lips may be difficult to achieve. All of his muscles tense when he moves, locking everything into one position, which could make his speech, sound like a stuttering block. In general, a cerebral palsied child can experience one or more of the following speech difficulties:[3]

- Pitch problems. There may be difficulties controlling the tone of voice. The voice can range wildly from a falsetto to a bass.
- Loudness. The child may not be able to control the volume of the voice. Or the child may not be able to sound the voice at all.
- Quality of voice. The voice may sound harsh or hoarse or breathy or nasal.
- Breathing control. The child may not be able to say as many syllables as normal on one breath and may need to pause at the wrong time to breathe in. This would result in a jerky rhythm of speech.
- Pronunciation. The child may lack the control of the speech organs to produce clear speech sounds. Chapter 5 has a complete discussion of this problem.
- Difficulty in being understood. With all or some of the above problems the child may be difficult to understand or may be totally unintelligible.
- "Different"-sounding speech. Even if the child can be completely understood the speech will sound odd to the listener's ear, which will interfere with communication.
- Language delay. Poor vocabulary and grammar from language

3. E. D. Mysak, "Cerebral Palsy," from *Human Communication Disorders*, ed. by G. Shames and E. Wiig (Columbus, OH: Charles E. Merrill Publishing Company, 1982). Seventy to 86 percent of children with cerebral palsy have communication disorders. Why should speech be so vulnerable to this type of brain damage? Almost half of the brain's sensory and motor control centers are dedicated to the oral speech organs. This brain space reflects the complexity of the system rather than its overall size. But the chance of affecting motor speech control is great.

delay resulting from mental retardation or unstimulating environment. Chapter 3 discusses this problem in detail.

Problems of Evaluation of a Cerebral Palsied Child

There is always the question of intellectual development with a
child like Luis. Some think that cerebral palsy affects intelligence
as well as the ability to move. There are certainly cases in which
there is intellectual impairment. But one should not automatically
assume the worst. Luis's parents may want to have their son tested
for intellectual potential, but how *can* he be tested? The intelligence tests given to young children examine motor and speech
development as indicators of intelligence. Luis's parents know
without going to a specialist that Luis falls below normal in these
areas. Later in the preschool years intelligence tests have verbal
items requiring spoken response and performance items, requiring
the child to do something like putting together a puzzle. The testing methods we have available are probably not adequate to assess
intelligence in children like Luis, with abilities which we know are
impaired. Moreover, the confinement experienced by children like
Luis, and their physical dependency, create an unstimulating environment which in itself shows up in lower IQ scores. Most developmental tests including the IQ tests are designed to predict the
child's ultimate intellectual achievement. I really do not think it is
possible for a moderately to severely impaired cerebral palsied
child to be tested this way. It *is* possible to assess what Luis can do
at any given time without any predictive judgment. The examiner
could assess Luis's speech and language understanding skills at the
present through sensitive and careful testing by establishing
enough rapport with the child to develop a system of communication. For example, if a severely impaired child could indicate understanding by blinking the eyes, the sensitive examiner would use
this method to measure language understanding. Most predictive
standardized tests do not allow such leeway in type of response.

Help for the Cerebral Palsied Child

Since Luis's problems cover so many disabilities he needs a team of
professionals to help him with his development and habilitation.
Luckily the local university medical center has a physical therapy

clinic which uses this team approach to cerebral palsied patients. First Luis was sent to a neurologist who confirmed the pediatrician's diagnosis. The neurologist acted as the coordinator of Luis's therapy team and emphasized to the parents that the various therapists on the team would instruct them how to teach and help their child. There would be physical therapy to help Luis learn coordinated movements. There would be occupational therapy to help Luis take care of himself in the everyday world. There would be an orthopedist (specialist in disorders of the skeletal system) to help Luis overcome physical problems brought on by the motor disabilities. Another member of the team was a clinical psychologist with a double task: to assess Luis's intellectual capacity as accurately as possible and to help Luis's parents bring up their "different" child. Even before Luis was ready to talk the parents needed a speech/language pathologist. They all anticipated that Luis would have trouble speaking clearly, but the speech/language pathologist wanted to make sure that Luis got a chance to develop his language as normally as possible. There would also be an audiologist to give Luis a complete hearing examination. Since 5 to 10 percent of cerebral palsied children have impaired hearing, Luis would be considered a high-risk child for hearing disorders. Chapter 4 has a thorough discussion of hearing problems in children. Later on more professionals would be added to the team, especially those in special education.

If Luis had not been so fortunate as to live near such a university medical center, his parents would have had to put together a habilitation team themselves. It would not have been the formal arrangement found in the medical center, but they would still have needed each of these professionals. They would have had the task of encouraging communication between the various specialists to coordinate their efforts in treating Luis.

Teaching Parents to Teach the Child

A problem encountered by cerebral palsied children learning to talk is that their brain function is immature. This interferes with their ability to control their bodies, especially the parts that produce speech. They often do not grow out of some infantile reflexes (such as rooting for a nipple when the cheek is touched, a response found in normal young babies). To combat this type of reflex, when it would interfere with a desired movement, the reflexive response is prevented by physical restraint. These physical therapy techniques are not only valuable for general motor development but have direct impact upon speech development. Before children can learn to speak they must hold up their head and trunk and must be able to move their jaws and tongues independently. Such physical training must be done by parents under the guidance of a professional physical therapist working on the team with the speech/language pathologist.

A physical therapist showed Luis's parents how to neutralize some of the primitive reflexes which get in the way of more controlled movements. While they manipulated the parts of Luis's body into desired movement patterns, at the same time discouraging undesirable patterns), they would talk and sing. The speech/language clinician told them that Luis would be more responsive to musical rhythm. So while they had him move his foot in and out, they made a little song about it and used words describing the parts of his body and what they were doing. Their technique was done to the tune of "Here we go loopty-loo, I put my right foot in, I put my right foot out, I give my right foot a shake shake shake and put it back again." This can be modified to fit all parts of the body. The musical accompaniment, with lyrics, made the exercises more fun for Luis and his parents and the technique also taught him the names of the parts of his body and the words for what he was doing.[4]

Teaching the Child to Listen and Look

Luis was easier to handle in many ways than most babies because he was not always getting into things. Friends would tell the parents about the "terrible twos," but at two years Luis did not get into trouble, not because he was more virtuous, but because he couldn't. Normal children often drive their parents to distraction, but that exploration is the way small children learn. Without the mobility to explore, the ability to learn about the world is curtailed

---

4. Various physical therapy programs are designed to free the speech articulators from extraneous movements which hinder speech. Among them are the Bobath method, which inhibits abnormal reflexes by physical restraint once the reflex is stimulated. Another is the Rood technique, which uses various different objects to stimulate the skin—ice, brushes, etc.—training relaxation.

and often stunted. Luis's parents had to bring the world to Luis. Instead of simply feeding him, they would tease him a little with the food before they let him eat it. In this way he would become aware of it and what it was. They would let him smell the peach before they let him eat it. By allowing him the pleasures of antici- pation, he would have the chance to think the word as well as experience the object. Before Luis could sit up alone they propped him into a sitting position so that he could see what was going on. To teach Luis to clap, one or the other parent would first take his hands and bring them together, making sure he could see them. Then they would bring his hands together hard enough to make a sound. Soon they were helping Luis clap to the rhythm of music. They wanted him to respond actively to rhythm. They were pleased when they realized that Luis was not depending very much upon their manipulation of his hands in order to clap. *He* was doing it himself. Then they added some nonsense words to his routine. After a while Luis was clapping to music and singing *bah bah bah* in time. Whenever his movements became disorganized one of his parents would gently guide him. Games that were suc- cessful started out with a single activity such as the clapping; then they added one activity at a time, the music and then the syllables. If his parents had tried all three from the beginning Luis would have had a harder time.

In order to stimulate Luis to use his tongue, his parents would smear a tiny dab of peanut butter on a spot near or even in Luis's mouth. Thus motivated, he would find the spot with his tongue. Before the peanut butter trick, Luis had not been able to put his tongue tip on the corner of his mouth when asked to copy the action.

Luis's parents wanted to make sure their son learned to listen to different sounds. They realized that it is easy for a normal child to check out an unfamiliar sound. But if Luis heard something he did not understand, he would have no way of finding out about it unless someone helped him find the source of what he was hear- ing. If a person is surrounded constantly by sights and sounds that can't be understood, that person gives up trying to make sense out of them and so does not learn from them. His parents wanted to help Luis understand the sounds around him, especially the sounds of talking. They would use two different-sounding toys when they played with him. After having sounded the rattle and the bell in

Luis's sight so that he could see which one was making what noise, a parent would shake one or the other out of the child's sight. Then the parent would reveal both toys. If Luis looked toward the toy he had heard the parent would smile and tell him what a smart boy he was. When Luis was in his crib, the parents would speak to him from different parts of the room in order to give him awareness of different directions. During their sound games Luis's parents realized that Luis's hearing seemed good enough to understand speech. They felt better knowing that even if Luis were never able to speak clearly, there was no reason he could not understand clearly.

Giving the Child the Experience Which Stimulates Language

Luis's parents not only were able to enrich his world with stimulating sights and sounds but they worked upon enriching his sense of touch and temperature. A child who is confined by a motor disability may not experience the many differences in texture and climate. The parents took him outside in the winter to experience the feeling of chill air on his face. They let him play with warm water and then changed it to cool water so he could feel the contrast. They gave him sand to play in, also pebbles and larger rocks. Every time they gave Luis a new touch experience, they would talk about it in simple terms, giving him the words to go with what he was feeling.

Some of the activities that Luis and his parents did were suggested by the speech pathologist. The parents, however, wanted to do more and expand their training program. Therefore they looked at normal children and what they were doing at Luis's developmental stage (not necessarily his chronological age). They observed that other babies reached out for objects and put them in their mouths and understood that this taste-testing of objects was part of a child's learning procedure. Realizing that Luis would have difficulties in coordinating his movements well enough to put things into his mouth, and not wanting him to miss out on this almost universal experience, the parents placed safe toys in Luis's mouth so that he could feel and taste them. Some people believe that the ability to identify objects in the mouth is related to speaking skill, so Luis's parents wanted this kind of mouth experience for their son, which they felt would enhance his speech. Friends

and family disapproved. Nevertheless Luis's parents were convinced that normal children have their own learning "agenda,"
parts of which are often annoying to their parents but necessary to
children's development into thinking human beings. So despite
feeling a little silly doing it, they put blocks and balls into their
son's mouth.[5]

Relaxation

As Luis grew older it became pretty clear to his parents that he
understood what was being said. But his own speech attempts were
not successful. When the parents brought Luis to the speech clinic,
they realized the power of the team approach. The speech pathologist and the physical therapist worked together to help Luis learn
to speak. Luis's problem was not that he had too little muscle
activity but too much. Whenever he tried to move or do something, too many muscles would be brought into play, making
movements which prevented him from speaking. The physical
therapist taught Luis's parents exercises for their son designed to
help him relax his muscles, to give him the control to turn muscles
off so that he could make gentle movements without hindrance.
The physical therapist and the speech pathologist found that Luis
could make speech movements better if he were making chewing
motions at the same time. The chewing motions seemed to use up
the excess muscle activity that so often stood in the way of speech
but they did not really interfere with it. (Parents of normal children know all too well that it is possible to talk and chew at the
same time.) The physical therapist and the speech pathologist also
worked on Luis's breathing pattern, which had been one of taking
many short shallow breaths, none of which provided him with a
large enough air supply to last more than two syllables. By learning to breathe more slowly and deeply, Luis gradually built up his
breath power and could lengthen his speaking. The new way of

5. J. E. Bernthal and N. W. Bankson, *Articulation Disorders* (Englewood Cliffs, NJ:
Prentice-Hall, 1981). Oral form recognition has been thought by researchers to have a
relationship with speech skill because speaking involves sensory feedback of the speech
organs. The results from the experiments to demonstrate this relationship are inconsistent
and inconclusive. Yet children *do* put things in the mouth and just because the experiments have failed to demonstrate the relationship does not necessarily mean there isn't
any.

breathing helped Luis to be more relaxed, which in turn also helped his speech.

Allowing the Child Some Independence

The speech/language pathologist admired all the things that Luis's parents had done to bring the world to Luis so that he would have as normal as possible experiences. But perhaps the parents were doing too much. Sometimes it is necessary for a child to explore on his own. It is impossible to bring the whole world into the reach of a small child. The act of reaching out may itself be a necessity. At four years old Luis finally learned to walk. His gait was lurching, however, and he always walked on the balls of his feet. His parents were fearful for his safety and discouraged him from moving around on his own. They were afraid to let Luis climb stairs or play in the playground and were beginning to communicate their fears to him. The cerebral palsy team at the medical center tried to advise them to let Luis experience physical risks of falling down so that he could learn to move as independently as possible. The speech/language pathologist saw that confinement of Luis's physical world would slow down his language development. They tried to persuade his parents to let him move around to increase his walking, speech and language development. The clinical psychologist on the team counseled his parents on how to stop being "overprotective." They compared the physical risks of allowing Luis to move independently (within reason) to the psychological risks of making Luis more dependent and more handicapped than he needed to be. It was a difficult time. Every mother and father can understand what pain Luis's parents felt as they watched him lurch toward the slide on the playground, scramble up the ladder, finally make it to the top, teetering and giving every expectation of tumbling to the hard ground below, and finally sitting on the slide and sliding down. When Luis's mother and father talked about this to other parents they realized that they all feared for the safety of their children and had to suppress the desire to overprotect. They watched while a neighbor's normal seven-year-old rode his two-wheel bicycle down the street for the first time. They saw another's teenage daughter drive the family car alone for the first time. These youngsters' parents were extremely anxious about their children's safety but felt it was necessary to their children's growth to develop into responsible indepen-dent people. So Luis's parents crossed their fingers, held their breath and let their child explore on his own. There were cuts and bruises, but there was also a more lively little boy. As Luis ven-tured out on his own he found more to talk about and stretched his language more and more. When Luis was six years old he came lurching and stumbling in from outside full of talk and excitement. Luis's mother went out into the yard to see what he was talking about and found an injured bird. Luis had saved it from a neigh-borhood cat. He wanted to keep it so it could get well. Luis talked in long sentences for the first time. He really needed to communi-cate. Not only because he was excited at finding and rescuing the bird, but now he wanted something he was not sure his mother would let him have. Her first impulse was to let the bird alone and let nature take its course with it. But when she saw how much and how well Luis was talking about it she saw the bird as an opportu-nity instead of a nuisance. They took the bird inside, made it a bed from a shoebox, fed it some bread crumbs and put it in a safe place on the porch. When Luis's father came home the child had to tell him all about "my bird." The frustrations of coordinating his movements to form the words were momentarily forgotten in the desire to communicate. After a few days the bird disappeared from its box, cured and presumably well enough to join its flock. But the bird stayed on as a topic of conversation for some months. Even the speech pathologist was charmed with the story when Luis related it in great detail at the next session.

Accepting a Different-Sounding Child

As Luis grew his speech became clearer. His parents came to realize that it would never really sound normal, but it could be understandable. He talked more slowly than most people because the effort of coordinating his speech movements was still consider-able. He was encouraged to use the slower speech rate in order to give himself time to form the words. He is still not always in control of his voice. Sometimes he speaks in a high-pitched voice and at other times a low voice. But the most startling thing about his speech is that it will suddenly burst out after a blocked silence. His friends have become used to this blurting speech. Although obviously crippled, Luis is lucky. He can get around on his own and he can talk to other people. His accomplishments are largely due to his parents' effort.

The Nontalker

Joyce is fifteen years old. She was born with cerebral palsy. Her motor impairment is more severe than Luis's, and she is unable to walk or talk. Perhaps if she had been given intensive stimulation in the early years as Luis had, her physical disability would not be so severe. On the other hand the damage might have been too great for much physical habilitation. Joyce cannot control either of her hands or arms but she can control her head movements. Her main speech problem is that she cannot coordinate her outgoing breath with her voice box. Sometimes you can see her mouth the words but nothing comes out that anyone can understand. She is intellectually capable of communication and can understand all the speech around her. Joyce is one of the one and a half million nonspeakers in the United States.

These nonspeakers include people with severe cerebral palsy, or other neurological disorders (stroke victims and certain neurological diseases), severe structural deformities that make speech impossible, such as radical surgery of the lower face, and those who have lost their voices due to removal of the larynx (voice box). The last three groups of people usually have enough control over their bodies to make some sort of manual communication a possible alternative for speech. These nontalkers also include those who suffer from severe retardation and cannot learn to speak. Joyce is one of the nontalkers who want to speak, have something to say and understand others. The attempts to teach her to speak, however, have been abandoned. How can a nonspeaker communicate?

Alternative Communication Devices

Fortunately for Joyce, she is living at a time in which there has been much effort and progress in developing alternate forms of communication for people who cannot speak. The obstacles are great. The cerebral palsied do not usually find sign language any easier than speech because it also requires controlled movements. Moreover, most people do not know sign language. So although it has worked for some cerebral palsied individuals, sign language is not the best alternative means of communication. There are various communication boards by which the "speaker" can indicate the message simply by pointing. These vary in complexity from the simple homemade object board to communicate basic needs to electronically automated message boards. As a child Joyce started out with a homemade picture board, one with pictures placed in front of her on her wheelchair. The simple pictures represented basic needs such as a glass of water or a toilet. She had a pointer attached to a headband, and by moving her head could point to a picture and make a simple request. Later, as she learned to read, the board became a spelling board. It had all the letters and a few common words so that Joyce was able to communicate much more. Joyce's parents were glad to be able to communicate with their daughter and thought the communication was an answer to their difficulties. The problem with the spelling board is that it is slow and the "listener" has to pay constant attention. Communication is so tedious and cumbersome that you don't engage in small talk. Now, however, there are automated spelling boards, which are more versatile and faster, sometimes using a more streamlined symbol system than traditional writing.[6] Joyce's communication possibilities have expanded greatly with her microprocessor. She can activate it with a switch which can be controlled with a head movement. It is also less obtrusive than the head-band pointer apparatus. Joyce is experimenting with some of the new coding systems that make communication even smoother and faster. Computer technology is able to give nontalkers the ability to "talk." Joyce is now looking forward to having a synthetic voice. Instead of the listener having to read the messages Joyce wants to send, she will activate a speech synthesizer and she will have an actual voice. At the present, the quality of the voice is poor, but this technology is improving rapidly. Joyce expects some day soon to be able to speak electronically to a listener who will hear what she says expressed in an almost normal-sounding voice.[7]

6. Blissymbol communication is a system of symbols standing for whole ideas or concepts rather than single words or letters. On a communication board they would be considerably faster.

7. For children who can speak but not always intelligibly, there are several forms of modified speech: the child can identify the topic as a comprehension aid; the child can spell the word which is not understood. Electronic devices can filter and amplify the child's own speech to make it clearer.

Social Problems Encountered by the Nontalker

Joyce feels that speaking with a voice, even a synthesized voice, will help her overcome the social problems encountered by those who cannot talk. Many people who see a nontalker for the first time assume that the nontalker is stupid (dumb). Even when Joyce's family tried to assure strangers that Joyce was not retarded they would still treat her that way—much to her dismay and frustration. One nontalker wryly remarks that he should work for the FBI or the CIA because people carry on confidential conversations in his presence as if he could not understand them. Another frustrating thing about being a nontalker is that people do not talk back to you. Joyce has found that people whisper to her or they keep their sentences very simple as if they were talking to a two-year-old. Joyce has come to feel that many of her problems are created by other people. She is disabled, but other people make her disability worse. Joyce's parents have become active in educating the public about the problems of the handicapped, especially the communicatively handicapped. There is a two-pronged effort on the behalf of the nontalking population. Public awareness and acceptance of alternative methods of communication form one approach.[8] Electronic technology to create a natural-sounding voice and methods to program the voice to say what the person wants to say form the other. Although Luis's parents did not need to explore alternative methods of communication for their son, it was some comfort to them, when they wondered whether Luis would ever talk clearly enough, to know that there were other methods available.

The Clumsy Child: A Mild Case of Cerebral Palsy

George at ten years old seems a normal child. He keeps up with his classmates at school and seems a happy and outgoing boy. But he always is wearing a bandage and several Band-Aids to cover the innumerable bruises on his body. He falls down stairs, he falls off bicycles, he trips over obstacles, he bumps into things. All this in spite of repeated requests from parents and teachers to watch

8. R. Creech and J. Viggiano, "Consumers Speak Out on the Life of the Non-speaker," *Asha*, vol. 23, no. 8, 1981. Two extremely articulate accounts by nonspeakers who are helping to perfect electronic communication aids.

where he is going. When it is time to choose up teams at recess, George is the last to be chosen. The team captain only takes him with extreme reluctance because George can be counted on to drop the ball instead of catch it or fall down instead of run. Nevertheless, although thought of as "klutzy," George is not considered handicapped. George was slow at learning to talk clearly and still does not speak as precisely as other children. Some of his clumsiness was in his mouth, and his speech was slurred and mumbled during his kindergarten and early grades. He had speech therapy in school which made it easier to understand him. Because the school clinician felt that George's speech was clearer when it was slow, he was encouraged to speak more slowly than normal. The clinician could not teach George to speak clearly at a normal rate. During an examination of his mouth, the clinician noticed a faint tremor in George's jaw. The tremor was not repeated and no further examination was made. George's speech problem was attributed to slow learning of speech sounds, a very common problem with children.

What George's parents and teachers do not know is that George, like Joyce and Luis, has cerebral palsy. It is so mild that no one realizes it. This is one of the cases of cerebral palsy which never gets counted. George's pediatrician has considered the possibility of brain damage accounting for his slow speech development and clumsiness while treating the boy often for a series of cuts, bruises, sprains, and broken bones. But the boy is living a normal life and doing well. Since cerebral palsy is a condition which does not get worse with time, and for which there is no cure, the doctor felt that there was no point in alerting the parents to the possibility that George might be mildly affected.

George's parents have noticed, however, that George's speech is more difficult to understand when he is tired. They have also noticed that it takes longer for George to learn a new skill such as tying knots or writing than it seems to take with other children. They are patient with him, attributing his difficulties to the normal differences among people. It is perhaps best for George that no one has labeled him as having cerebral palsy and that there is no need for him to think of himself as disabled. He can and is making it without special help. (On the other hand it was very important for Luis that his parents were aware of the condition early so that they could give him the extra help he needed.) Perhaps George would have benefited from early help. But he might have lost out too. His parents, believing he was handicapped, might not have let him ride his bicycle and expose himself to the bumps and bruises of the world. It may be that his normal language and his almost normal speech are a result of his launching himself into a normal boy's life.[9]

There is no way to know how many children like George there are. Where does one draw the line between clumsiness and motor disability? There are many people who cannot become great athletes and there are many people who cannot become radio or TV announcers. The best thing that parents can do is to accept their children, their talents and inabilities. George's parents accepted George and were not disappointed when he did not star on the playing field or in the school play.

Cerebral Palsy Covers a Wide Range of Handicapping Conditions

Luis, Joyce and George illustrate the wide variation of severity of motor disability included in the term "cerebral palsy." There are many other cerebral palsied children who have very different disabilities. Many of the children are multiply handicapped, their motor problems being complicated by additional problems of poor vision, hearing loss, perceptual deficits and mental retardation. Sometimes the abnormal movement patterns cause a limb to be deformed. Even if the speaking itself were not affected such children would have communication problems. Still speech is often impaired because talking is an activity requiring fine muscle control, the major problem for people with cerebral palsy.

There are many people moderately or severely affected with cerebral palsy who are living normal and satisfying lives in spite of their disability. More and more public places and schools are building in accessibility for people with motor handicaps. There are adults at the present who did not go to high school, not because they could not do the academic work, but because the only high school in their locality had too many steps to climb. The critical

9. George was mildly affected by cerebral palsy and also did not suffer one of the accompanying conditions. Probably some cases of minimal brain dysfunction, perceptual disorders and learning disabilities are "subclinical" cases of cerebral palsy. Early understanding of the true nature of the disorder would be helpful in such cases.

factor for the person with cerebral palsy, however, is the ability to communicate with others. It is very hard to imagine a satisfying life cut off from human contact. The persons most responsible for the ability to communicate are the parents of the cerebral palsied child. Whenever I see a competent functioning cerebral palsied person, I know that the parents and the family were the ones responsible for the success. They worked, they taught, they supported, they loved—day in and day out. It is they who were the habilitation team.

Suggestions for the Parents of Children with Cerebral Palsy

Since there is such a wide range of conditions, it is impossible to present a typical case of cerebral palsy (Luis was possibly the most "typical") or present general guidelines. Therefore some of these suggestions may be applicable and helpful to your cerebral palsied child and some not.

- Be aware of high-risk situations which may be part of your child's prenatal or perinatal history. These include viral diseases during pregnancy, other pregnancy complications, delivery complications, head injury to the young baby. Discuss these factors with your doctor.
- Don't assume that the diagnosis of cerebral palsy means a helpless or hopeless cripple.
- Understand that the diagnosis of cerebral palsy means that you will have to make more than the usual parental effort to help your child's development.
- Try to get your child entered in a team remediation program. The problems are so varied no one professional has all the expertise necessary to treat your child.
- If you cannot find a rehabilitation center in your community, create your own team. You can get referrals to the various specialists you need: neurologist, orthopedist, speech/language pathologist, audiologist, physical therapist, psychologist etc. and coordinate them yourself by encouraging them to communicate with one another.
- Become aware of your school system's facilities for teaching the motorically handicapped and the communicatively disabled. Chapter 9 discusses your child's rights to an appropriate education.
- Contact the local chapter of the United Cerebral Palsy Association or the Association for Retarded Citizens or the Easter Seal Society. These groups offer the best sources of local information and resources. You

can find the local chapters through the phone book or by contacting the national organizations (see Organizations for Further Information, pp. 258–260).

- Realize that you will have to bring the world to your child because your child cannot reach out for experience alone.
- Realize that you will be the chief therapist for your child under professional guidance.
- Understand the difficulty in testing and evaluating your child.
- Don't try to predict the final outcome of your child's communication skills. Just keep trying for as much as possible.
- Be realistic and accept that your child probably will not ever sound normal.
- Realize that brain-injured children tire more quickly than normal children and your child will talk and perform much better when rested.
- Allow your child as much independence as possible.

8

If You Think Your Child Stutters: Changing Your Attitudes to Help Your Child to Fluent Speech

- *What Is Stuttered Speech?*
- *Who Are the Stutterers?*
- *Stuttering Starts with Normal Disfluency*
- *How Childish Disfluency Turns into True Stuttering*
- *How Stuttering Is Maintained: The Child Internalizes the Problem*
- *Other Beliefs about the Cause of Stuttering*
- *Stuttering Gets Worse or Better in Certain Situations*
- *The Difference Between Fluency Devices and Stuttering Cure*
- *Long-Term Stuttering Remedies*
- *Speech Therapy for Stuttering*
- *Dos and Don'ts for Parents of Disfluent Children*

Thirteen-year-old Bryan is in his room reading a book. He hears the telephone ring. It rings again. And again. Why doesn't somebody answer it? he wonders. Bryan realizes that he has to answer it, and his scalp begins to tingle. He moves toward the still-ringing phone and his hands begin to sweat. As his hand reaches for the receiver, his throat feels choked. His mouth goes dry and he runs out of air as he tries to say hello. All that comes out of Bryan's mouth is a strangled gasp. The voice at the other end says, "Who is this?" Bryan tries to identify himself. He closes his lips to start the word *Bryan*, but they lock up tight. No matter how much effort he makes, his name remains stuck somewhere in his throat. His face feels hot and flushed. After what seems to be a near eternity of superhuman effort he says, "B-b-b-b-b . . . ryan."

Sixteen-year-old Marilyn is in the local fast-food restaurant craving a hamburger with mustard and tomato. The waitress says, "What'll it be?" Marilyn says, "One hamburger with mmmmmmmmm. . . ." Her face reddens and her eyes are tightly shut. She clenches her fists and starts over, "One hamburger with t-t-t-t-t-ch. . . ." The waitress sighs and shrugs: "Y' want cheese?" Marilyn says, "Yes and mmmmmmmmmm . . ." The exasperated waitress completes the order herself, saying, "OK, cheese and mayonnaise." Marilyn nods and accepts the order she didn't want because it is too hard for her to say what she really wants.

What Is Stuttered Speech?

Bryan and Marilyn are stutterers or stammerers (the two words are interchangeable, Americans preferring the word stutterer and the British preferring stammerer). The sounds of the names themselves seem to express the problem. Many children and some adults do not talk smoothly. They make great efforts to say simple words; they repeat the word or the first part of the word, (such as *b-b-b-b-boy*) and sometimes they do not seem able to get the word out at all. They start to speak and then their mouths lock up so that no sound at all comes out in spite of their obvious struggle. Stutterers look as if they are fighting with their own mouths in a battle to speak. The whole process is so tiring, painful and tense that the stutterer tries to avoid talking whenever possible.

Stutterers say that they feel as though their tongues get glued to the roofs of their mouths, or that their throats close off so that the words get stuck in their chests. The harder they try to speak, the worse the stuttering becomes and the harder they have to try in order to speak. The stammerer's discomfort is communicated to the listener and often the listener tries to avoid listening or tries to help the stutterer out of the predicament by finishing the sentence or by diverting attention. Stutterers are so acutely aware of the listeners' negative reactions that they usually cannot bear to look at them—they look anywhere except at the person they are talking to.

Sometimes stutterers grimace in grotesque ways as they are trying to talk. They blink their eyes, stamp their feet, tap their fingers, pull out their hair, bang their heads, while they are trying to force the words out of their mouths. People who stutter are more miserable than we nonstutterers can ever imagine. Because they feel isolated by their lack of ability to talk easily, many choose careers which they believe will not require much talking. Often their social life is extremely limited. They suffer a great deal of anxiety in anticipating commonplace speech situations such as buying a pair of shoes or ordering a meal in a restaurant. Calling a plumber on the phone can cause as much stage fright as we would feel having to address an audience of hundreds. The affliction can disappear, however, when talking to the family dog or to a baby only to reappear when talking to a friend or a stranger. In most cases the stutterer is perfectly normal physically. The doctor cannot find any medical cause for the stuttering. In fact, aside from the pained and peculiar speech there is no way to tell a stutterer from a nonstutterer. The "glue" in the mouth, the "lump" in the throat and the "knot" in the chest stutterers feel are manifestations of their anxieties about speaking and have no physical basis whatsoever.

Who Are the Stutterers?

This mysterious ailment, stuttering or stammering, affects about 1 percent of people in the modern industrialized nations.[1] About 80 percent of the children who stutter seem to outgrow the affliction; the rest continue to suffer as adults. Therefore the incidence of stuttering is higher in children than adults. It affects more boys than girls. Some surveys have found the proportion of males to females as high as nine to one; others say it is four to one. But all the surveys agree that stuttering is far more prevalent among men and boys than among women and girls. There is no accepted explanation for the sex difference in prevalence of stuttering, although there have been some speculations.[2] It is also not clear why

1. Like all disorder prevalence statistics, this must be taken with a grain of salt. Different surveys have different definitions of stuttering (how severe it must be to be counted) and different ways of determining stuttering (ask the subject, ask the subject's parents, ask teachers). If the 1 percent figure is correct, there are more than 2 million stutterers in the United States.

2. Among the speculations for the sex difference in prevalence of stuttering are: boys are more pressured to perform well by their parents; girls are normally more verbal and therefore don't have as much normal disfluency as boys; male children show a higher incidence of many behavioral and physical disorders. These have not been proven and perhaps never could be proven. The female stutterer is not so rare, however; I have treated several.

some children outgrow stuttering without treatment and others do not.

Although industrialized countries as different culturally as Japan and Sweden show the same proportions of their populations as stutterers, the incidence of stuttering has been reported to vary widely among nonindustrialized peoples.[3] The Utes and the Shoshone Indians have no stuttering; their languages don't even have a word for it. Some cultures in Africa have a rate of stuttering three times greater than the United States. Some speech experts have reported cultural differences in types of stuttering; for example, the black stutterer tends to have long nonaudible hesitations while the white stutterer is more likely to repeat words, parts of words and phrases.[4]

Stuttering has been with the human race for a long time. Archaeologists have uncovered and translated a four-thousand-year-old carved stone inscription in a long dead language bearing a prayer to the gods to relieve the "poor wretch" of the unbearable impediment of tongue, a prayer surely uttered by many stutterers today. Moses had so much trouble speaking that he had his friend and associate Aaron do his speaking for him. Demosthenes overcame his affliction by learning to talk with his mouth full of pebbles. He became one of the greatest orators of ancient Greece. King Charles I of England was a stutterer and so was his descendant, King George VI of Britain.[5]

Stutterers are often intelligent ambitious people whose language and thinking processes are in no way as tangled and disorganized as their tongues. A stutterer may be able to write a message eloquently and elegantly and yet may not be able to read the writing aloud without stumbling and struggling. Lewis Carroll,

3. There have been speculations that stuttering occurs more frequently in some ethnic groups, especially in families whose ambitions are to be realized by the accomplishments of their children. Second-generation boys from European Jewish families are a good example. It is not known whether there is really a greater incidence of stuttering among this group.

4. O. Taylor, "Language Differences," from *Human Communication Disorders: An Introduction.* Ed. by G. H. Shames and E. Wiig (Columbus, OH: Charles E. Merrill Publishing Co. 1982). Black stutterers seem more successful at hiding their handicap, often by avoiding speech altogether and still maintaining a "cool" image.

5. The list of distinguished stutterers is long. Virgil, Newton, and Darwin were stutterers: this should be enough to demonstrate that stuttering is *not* from lack of intelligence.

whose mastery and control of the language is evident in every page of *Alice in Wonderland* and *Through the Looking Glass*, was a stutterer.

Stuttering tends to run in families, leading some to think it is inherited. Others say that it runs in families because of family attitudes about speech. But if one child in the family is a stutterer it is not likely that another child will stutter.

Stuttering Starts with Normal Disfluency

When children begin to speak they do not have the normal fluency of adult speech. This is a normal part of learning to talk. During this stage a child stumbles over speech the way a baby stumbles while learning to walk. When speaking, a child may hesitate, repeat or prolong sounds or parts of words and have generally jerky-sounding speech. The child is not aware that there is anything wrong and accepts the disfluencies as part of being little. All children go through this stage. The development of stuttering at this point depends entirely upon others' reactions to these speech mistakes. When some parents hear breaks in rhythm which sound similar to the breaks of rhythm they have heard from authentic stutterers, they are too quick to label these early normal disfluencies as stutters, and believe that their child has a problem when none actually exists. They have unrealistic expectations about how well or smoothly their child can talk at the preschool time of life, and do not accept these breakdowns as normal.

Some parents find it hard to believe that a child experiencing so much difficulty getting words out could possibly be unaware of it. Not only do preschool "stutterers" seem unaware of how tangled their speech is, they cheerfully accept it and do not try to avoid or fix it. It is only when parents and teachers point it out that the children realize they have a problem. When they work to overcome it, it becomes worse, much to the dismay of both the child and the parents. There are many who say that a stutterer does not become a true stutterer until the problem is diagnosed and recognized to be a problem by the speaker as well as the listener. The labeling—especially the self-labeling—is the critical difference between a child who stumbles over words and a true stutterer. If that is the case, why does there need to be stuttering at all? If the true affliction can be avoided by not labeling the child, why give it a label? The vicious circle occurs because of and in spite of the parents' best intentions.[6]

Robert, age five, is at the zoo with his mother.

> ROBERT: I saw a b-b-big mmmmmmmmmonkey . . . not a mmmmmmmmmonkey big-g-g-er [so excited he can hardly speak]. It was b-b-b-big big.
>
> MOTHER: A chimpanzee?
>
> ROBERT: B-b-b-bigger aaaaaaa. . . .
>
> MOTHER: OK, calm down. A gorilla?
>
> ROBERT: Ye-ye-ye—ah ah ah ah g-g-goribba. . . .
>
> MOTHER [interrupting]: Now slow down and say it right.
>
> ROBERT: A a a a a g-g-g-g-gorrrrrrrrr. . . . I can't say it.
>
> MOTHER: Yes, you can, just think about what you are saying.
>
> ROBERT: A a a a ag. . . .
>
> MOTHER: For heaven's sake all you have to do is try harder.

Notice how Robert's speech got worse and worse. The scene could have gone a different way:

> ROBERT: I saw a b-b-big mmmmmmmmmmonkey . . . not a mmmmmmmonkey big-g-ger. It was b-b-big big big.
>
> MOTHER: Where?
>
> ROBERT [pointing]: There.
>
> MOTHER: Oh, that's a gorilla.
>
> ROBERT: A a a g-g-goribba?
>
> MOTHER: That's right, a gorilla.
>
> ROBERT: A a big gor . . . I still can't say it.
>
> MOTHER [pointing to the gorilla]: He can't either. I used to get messed up and say goribba too when I was a little girl.
>
> ROBERT: Ah ah ah ah big big gor*illa*.
>
> MOTHER: Great, you can help me if I mess up again.

The second time through the scene Robert's speech got better. Why are these scenes so different? Consider the first: Robert is very excited. His vocabulary is being stretched. Chimpanzee and gorilla are words that he knows but has not spoken himself. His mother does not share his excitement. She is intolerant of the

6. W. Johnson, *Stuttering and What You Can Do About It* (Minneapolis: University of Minnesota Press, 1961). Johnson, a pioneer in the modern understanding and treatment of stuttering, says that stuttering begins in the "ear of the listener" rather than the mouth of the speaker. But stuttering is developed when the listener accepts the diagnosis of the listener.

breakdown in smooth speech flow, a breakdown brought upon by both excitement and the unfamiliar words. She evidently expects perfect speech no matter what the circumstances. Since she is not particularly interested in the zoo she discounts Robert's excitement. Although he is aware of stumbling on his speech in the beginning, Robert doesn't seem to care. At first he forgives himself and is about to pass off the tongue tangling. But mother won't let it go. She feels that this is as good a time as any to say it right. She has unrealistic expectations of a child's speaking skill. She manages to let him know his speech is not right and that he should put more effort in it. She is probably displaying her customary attitude toward Robert's speech. Now mother doesn't really know *what* is wrong with Robert's way of talking, only that something *is* wrong.

She doesn't have a workable remedy for his speech so she advises him to slow down and try harder. How do you "try harder" in talking? If you are five years old, trying harder means to use more muscular force. If you can't move something you push harder. The trouble with speech is that there is very little force or strength required, so trying harder doesn't make any sense. Try speaking with greater muscular effort yourself. You will find it is possible only if you hold back your words to create a resistance to talking. Try to say the word *push* with greater effort. You need to clamp your lips tightly so that it takes more force from your breath stream to get out the rest of the word. You have to create an impediment to your speech in order for you to be able to exert extra muscular effort on it. Thus Robert, when he was told to try harder, held the back of his tongue tightly against the roof of his mouth, so tightly that he could not get past the G in *gorilla*. Robert also has no way of understanding what was wrong with his talking. He knows that there is *something* wrong and that it involves his mouth and throat because he knows where his words come from. So he becomes superconscious of his mouth and breathing, aware that there is a problem there somewhere. Not only is there a problem but it is so bad that his mother dislikes him for it. If he could talk better and try harder, maybe she would like him better. So he does try harder. Robert is not yet a stutterer, but he has a good chance of turning into one.

Now let us look at the second scene. First Robert's mother shares his excitement at the outing. Instead of talking, she indicates that she also wants to look. Robert does not have the tension of expressing his feelings to a resistant mother; she already shares them. Mother knows that the word *gorilla* is a new one and does not expect perfection right away—anyway, *goribba* was almost right. Mother hears the prolonged beginnings of words but does not pay any attention to it. Lots of children do that when they are keyed up. When Robert complains on his own that the word is unpronounceable, his mother acknowledges that it is a hard word with a little joke about how the gorilla himself can't say it and admits to having had trouble with it herself. Not only is Robert reassured that it is no big deal to stumble over words but even his mother has done it and needed help. Robert and his mother are sharing the experience of the zoo and even the difficult word together. From this background it is unlikely that Robert will turn into a full-fledged stutterer, even though his speech is jerky and nonfluent.

All children are nonfluent, some more than others. Some parents notice it but shrug it off as part of the difficulties their children encounter in learning to speak, just as they expect their children to fall down when they are learning to walk and run. Children often overshoot their ability to express ideas and thoughts and the words come tumbling out helter-skelter. The sense of balance and grace in children finally catches up to their locomotion plans. And when the ability of children to speak smoothly catches up to their ability to think of things to say, the disfluency is outgrown. It sometimes seems to take a long time for a child to choose the right words, put them into the correct order, pronounce them all correctly and maintain normal speaking rate and smooth rhythm. Some parents don't even notice their child's stumbling in speech, and that is fine as far as the child's fluency is concerned.

The Danger of Too Much Concern over a Child's Fluency

There are some parents, however, who become concerned because they do not realize how hard it is to develop a smooth flow of speech. They are too quick to label the little repetitions and hesitations as stuttering; in fact, they *do* sound like stuttering. Once they have said the word to themselves or to each other, all the negative images they have about stuttering haunt them and add to their worry and anxiety about their child. They have visions of their child suffering from what they know can be a crippling handicap and fear that their child's life will be limited and blighted by this affliction. Perhaps they know a stutterer or there is a stutterer in the family and so are very aware of the problem. Because they are so concerned, they pick up on every little break in speech they hear from their child and forget to listen for them in other children's speech or even their own. They communicate their concern to the child and thus set up the beginning of true stuttering.

After a while the child understands there is a problem because the parents *think* there is a problem, identifies it as not speaking smoothly and that it is called stuttering. As soon as the child recognizes this anxiety over speech, desire to avoid stuttering and dread of failure set in. Thus the problem created by parental worry over their (mistaken) diagnosis becomes one that the child must bear— worry about speech. Or put another way, the problem begun in the ear of the listener shifts to the mouth of the speaker. The true difference between normal disfluency and stuttering is not in the frequency and severity of the rhythm breaks but rather in the child's attempt to *avoid* these rhythm breaks. Since it is virtually impossible for anyone to avoid some rhythm breaks in speech, the attempt to avoid them is bound to fail. Each break in rhythm that the child is unable to avoid convinces that child that speech is disordered. The parents also become more and more convinced that their child's speech is defective because the problem seems to be getting worse. In addition to the normal disfluency, the child's attempts to avoid it show up as additional disfluency, because anything a child does to modify speech breaks the rhythm. For instance, if, as an aid in speaking, the child takes a deep breath before starting, that deep breath will be noticed as a peculiar speech pattern.

Fluency-Risk Situations for Your Child to Avoid

As a parent you are in a position to help avoid your child's becoming a stutterer even if that child is quite disfluent but does not yet realize it. You will want to understand the situations which are most apt to cause rhythm breakdown, keeping them in mind as you judge your child's speech. As we saw with Robert, a new and exciting situation, even one enjoyable to the child, leads to breaks in fluency. Another fluency-risk situation for a child is performing or reciting before a group, especially a group of adults or an unfamiliar adult. A third situation of fluency breakdown that children experience is competing to be heard. If the child is worried about being interrupted, to hold the floor there will be prolongations and fillers such as "well" and "you know" and "er," which can sound like stuttering.

Putting your child on the spot or being an interrogator is another tense speech situation which can lead to disfluency. Many times parents ask their children questions which they cannot or do not want to answer. Asking your child, "Who broke this plate?" has an accusatory ring to it. Even without knowing how the plate was broken, your child will feel defensive and pressured to prove innocence. Of course if your child really did break the plate, it will be hard to answer the question fluently. Sometimes children do not recognize that a rhetorical question doesn't need an answer and feel put on the spot. If you say upon finding the broken plate, "Now what do you think of that?" your child may think an answer is required and become tense in a speech situation.

Some parents might want to avoid these fluency-risk situations altogether. The disfluencies do not in themselves make stuttering but the attitude toward the disfluencies creates the stuttering. Consequently, parents might think that the less disfluency the child has, the less chance the stuttering pattern has to develop. It is not possible, however, to avoid all situations for your child which are apt to cause speech breakdowns. The parent can avoid some of the common mistakes in trying to remedy the speech breakdowns. Many well-meaning parents and relatives try to help by finishing the child's sentence, telling the child to slow down, or worse, telling the child to think carefully about how and what to say before starting. Sometimes the parents ask the child to start all over again and this time say it right.

Why You Should Not Help Your Child During the Disfluent Events

Why don't these remedies work? Imagine your own four-year-old child whom you ask to recite a nursery rhyme for all the relatives at a family reunion. You may not realize that the child can feel some anxiety about it just as you might feel if asked to speak before a large group. After some trouble getting started, the first line goes OK, but the beginning of the second line breaks

down. "Ssssssing a song of sixpence, P-p-p-p-p-p. . . ." Suppose
you finish the line in a desire to be helpful and minimize the
trouble. Your child would know not only that there was something
wrong with the delivery of the recitation, but that it was so bad
that you had to take the task away. The child would feel a failure.
It is very frustrating to have someone else snatch the words out of
your mouth just because they are not spoken fast enough. So you
would have added frustration and a sense of failure to the natural
stage fright of the situation. Finishing a sentence for your child is
definitely one response you should avoid.

Suppose you had told your child to take a deep breath and start
over? Again you would have judged the child's performance as
inadequate. You would have said in effect, "Say it over and say it
right this time." Your child wants to do it right but does not know
how. A mistake in speaking has been made. But what mistake?
Where? You can't correct a mistake unless you can locate it, identify it and know what the right way would be. So your child would
start over with no more idea of how to recite properly than the
first time, but this time knowing you were displeased.

Thus the two ways of helping would actually serve to hinder
the child's fluency. Moreover the child would see this as disapproval in general. Children take things very personally. Mistaken
speech in a child who is learning speech is not bad behavior and it
is unjust to penalize a child for it, especially when this penalty can
be interpreted as disapproval and dislike of the child as a person.

What Parents Can Do to Help Their Normally Disfluent Child

Rethink your speech standards to be realistic. What can you
do when your child's rhythm breaks down while reciting? Ignore
the breakdown and praise the speech. Why should this be hard?
You want your child to succeed. You want to be proud and show
off this marvelous and lovable child to your relatives. Your own
ego is involved here. You have to accept the idea that the standards of fluency for your four-year-old are different from the standards for you or even for an older child. The fact that your child
would recite at all is rather wonderful and should be regarded as
such. You may be worried about the opinion of others at the party,
but their opinion of your child's performance is not so important to

your child as is yours. Let the others think what they will; you should be proud and supportive of your child's speech, stumbles and all. You should not bring the breaks in rhythm to your child's attention. If you accept them casually, your child will accept them casually. Your child learns to judge events by observing your judgment. If you feel shame, your child sees that shame is the appropriate emotion under these circumstances and will feel shame also. If you feel your child has been successful, your child will feel successful.

It is not easy to change your own attitudes about speech. When you hear what sounds like stuttering in your own child it is natural that you want to do what you can to alleviate it. If you are like most people, you are made uncomfortable and embarrassed by listening to a true stutterer. This embarrassment will be communicated to your child unless you change your beliefs and attitudes about speech.

Listen to rhythm breaks in other people's speech. One thing that might help you be the supportive parent you want to be is for you to be able to put the disfluencies into perspective. Listen for the disfluencies in those with normal speech, in your own speech. You may be surprised to discover, after careful listening, that absolute fluency almost never happens. We are constantly pausing, adding fillers, hanging up on part of a word, interrupting ourselves and starting over. The reason you probably haven't noticed this before is that these disfluencies are passed over casually by both speaker and listener. When you become aware of all the disfluencies in normal speech, you will be able to take your child's speech breaks more easily. Listen, too, for all the fluencies in your child's speech. Chances are that the major part of your child's speech is smooth and fluent. In your worry you have focused on the mistakes and forgotten to listen to the good parts.

Analyze what you do when you stumble in talking. As you become aware of the disfluencies in your own speech, think of how you handle them. What do you do when you occasionally stumble over your words while talking? You probably correct yourself. If you make a mistake in speaking and point out the mistake to your child, you give the child a model of self-correction. For example, you could be talking about rivers and say, "The biggest river in the United States is the Mis-ti-pi—no, that's not right. Missssissippi, there, that's got it, Mi-ssi-ssi-ppi." You have accepted your own speech stumble easily and showed how you correct yourself. You communicate to your child both your method of self-correction and your easy emotional attitude toward it. Moreover, by accepting your own speech stumble easily, you communicate your acceptance of your child's speech stumbles. Thus you are preventing the development of the vicious circle of expectation of stuttering/ fear of stuttering/attempt to avoid stuttering/stuttering/expectation of stuttering.

Even if you do accept your child's disfluencies easily, you will still want to minimize the number of speech breaks by minimizing the number of tense speaking situations.

Don't interrupt your child while your child is trying to tell you something.

Don't finish your child's message. Even though you can anticipate what is going to be said, it is better to let the child complete the thought without help.

Really listen to your child. If a child gets the idea that your attention is wandering, tension over getting and keeping your attention will build.

Keep others listening. You can help in larger family groups in which your child may not be able to get a turn talking. You might try using your authority to help your child gain and maintain the floor for a turn at talking in the family gathering.

How Childish Disfluency Turns into True Stuttering

After this first stage of normal disfluency, which the child is unaware of or doesn't pay attention to, there is a second stage in the development of stuttering: that point when the child stumbles and breaks the rhythm of speech, knowing that there is some problem with speaking smoothly but not trying to avoid it. The child may already be labeled a stutterer but doesn't understand nor take the label to heart yet. Some parents of children in this stage say that the child stutters but is either unaware of it or doesn't seem to care about it.[7] Some parents even say that it is necessary to point out the

7. I feel that one explanation for the great number of children who stuttered and grew out of it without treatment is that many parents label the disfluencies as stuttering without attaching much significance to it, thinking that stuttering is something that a lot of children do and expecting them to grow out of it. Most of our documentation on these child stutterers who were not treated is from adults who remembered stuttering in their childhood.

VICIOUS CIRCLE OF STUTTERING

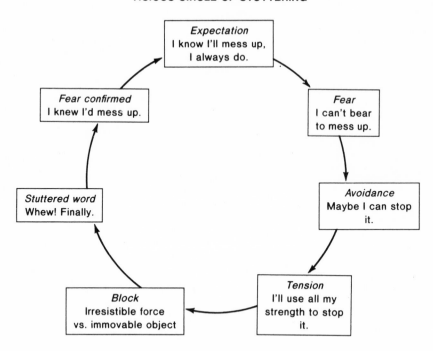

instances of stuttering to their child. Even at this stage, when your child is aware of not always being able to speak smoothly, there is still time to prevent the true pattern of stuttering from developing. Everything parents should do for their normally disfluent child should be done for their child who is beginning to be aware of the disfluencies: ignore breakdowns of speech rhythm in the child, self-correct breakdown in yourselves, do not call the rhythm breakdowns "stuttering," try to ease up on emotional pressure for the child, try to manipulate speaking situations as much as possible to avoid tension in speaking. Even with a child who is aware of disfluencies, the stuttering can be avoided if the child does not develop an emotional attitude toward speech rhythm.

Your child will pick up your emotional attitude; therefore, the place to start is with you. If you can believe that disfluencies in a child are not necessarily the beginning of stuttering then you do not have to fear them. You do not have to be embarrassed when your child stumbles while talking if you know that such stumbles are a natural part of growing up. In order to prevent stuttering

SIGNS OF STUTTERING

Unaware (first) stage	Prolongs some speech sounds.
	Repeats words or parts of words.
	Stumbles because speech is too rapid.
	Either unaware or unconcerned.
Emerging awareness (second) stage	Prolongs some speech sounds.
	Repeats words or parts of words.
	Long pauses.
	Uses fillers such as *well, er,* etc.
	Corrects speech easily after disfluency.
True stuttering pattern (third) stage	Prolongs some speech sounds.
	Repeats words or parts of words.
	Uses fillers such as *well, er,* etc.
	Long pauses.
	Evidence of inner struggle.
True stuttering pattern	Tries to avoid speaking.
	Uses circumlocutions to avoid feared word.
	Difficulty getting started talking.
	Gestures such as arm waving, hand or foot tapping, blinking, grimacing while trying to talk.
	Avoids looking directly at listener.
	Involuntary tremor of jaw or lip.

from developing you must prevent the child from feeling set apart from other people because of not being able to speak smoothly. When the child takes on the label and burden of being a stutterer, true stuttering begins. The child has anxieties about speech and fears a breakdown. From this point the parents' attitudes are secondary to the child's own attitude.

How Stuttering Is Maintained: The Child Internalizes the Problem

The Self-Fulfilling Prophecy

The parents' attitudes toward their children's speech may be what starts the stuttering in the first place. But what keeps it going? Once this third stage is reached, the parents' input is no longer necessary to maintain stuttering. Most of us have seen adults whose parents are far away or long dead who still stutter. Some adult stutterers seem to be worse than they were as children. The self-fulfilling prophecy is the simplest explanation: the person who stutters *expects* to stutter. Past experience makes that a reasonable prediction. If your child knows that a certain word will be difficult to say, anticipates not being able to say it and fears the inevitable speech block, when it comes time to say the dread word sure enough the mouth will tighten up and the speech apparatus will be unable to move. Then after a certain amount of struggle and effort, the terrible word is finally said. The next time a feared word is anticipated the child is even more sure that the attempt to say it will end up in a block. Now the child may be afraid of stuttering and wish to avoid it on the one hand, but on the other hand knows from past experience that the talking will eventually come after the block. A part of the stutterer's mind grows fond of the stutter, believing that without it speech would be impossible. You may see a child's speech improve a great deal after a bad stuttering block. Unfortunately such a "cure" is only temporary.

The Most Dangerous Word—the Stutterer's Own Name

The most difficult question for many stutterers to answer is "What's your name?" It is the question most often asked a child by strangers and also the one question you expect the person to be able to answer. Charles had trouble saying his name. It would sound like "Ch-ch-ch-ch-ch- . . . Charles." At school he had trouble with all the CH words such as *cheese, chip* and *choose*. When someone asked his name he would give a nickname, Tiny. He disliked the nickname, but it started with a safe sound, *T.* Sometimes he would answer the question with a high-speed running start almost as if he had to jump through it: "MynameisCh-Charles." When he grew up, Charles decided to change his name legally to Franklin. He had never had any trouble with the F. As soon as the judge signed the papers the Fs became impossible to say and when asked his name, he would hesitate, breathe deeply and say "FFFFFFFFFFFFFFFffffffffranklin." What Charles/Franklin did not realize was that there was nothing difficult about the word Charles in itself. What made it difficult to say was that it was *his* name, a word magically bound up with himself. A new name took on the same qualities the old name had and became the new stumbling block in speech.

When you ask a child, "What's your name?" you may think

you are merely being friendly, but you may actually be putting the child on the spot. You expect an answer and you expect it fast. The child who can't answer right off seems pretty dumb. The child knows this attitude and if fluency is a problem feels that the question is loaded. This may be the first time you notice a stutteringlike block in your child's speech. You are out with your child and someone asks "What's your name?" Wanting to help you may supply the name yourself or show your shame that the question seems too hard for your child to answer. Your task is not only to bear with the hesitation but act if it were perfectly normal. Your attitude will be communicated to the outsider as well as your child, and the stakes for failure can be lowered.

Helping the Child Who Has Internalized the Problem

Put fluency into perspective. All too often stutterers give their speech difficulties an unrealistic, often obsessive, place in their hierarchy of worries and it becomes the only problem they worry about. They think that if stuttering were solved they wouldn't have any other problems. I once asked a young man, "How would your life change if your stuttering suddenly disappeared?" He described a brilliant academic career at a prestigious four-year college instead of the two-year community college where he had gone. This would have been followed by graduate work in some highly technical field like computer science and then a lucrative and fascinating job. He thought all this would easily have happened if only he had fluent speech. In fact his financial situation was extremely limited, and his high school grades had been only fair in technical subjects. There were obviously many other barriers to his dream than speech, but speech was so all-important in his mind that he was unable to see them. As a parent you should make sure that you are not encouraging this disproportionate attitude. Try not to fall into believing that your child is or would be perfect except for this one affliction.

Just as parents of children going through a period of normal disfluency were advised earlier to listen to rhythm breaks in normal speech, parents of established stutterers should also listen critically to nonstuttering speech. You and your child can do this together. Once you start looking for them you can find them everywhere. One mother was astonished when she realized that her sister who did not stutter actually had more breaks in her speech than her daughter who did stutter. Neither she nor her sister had ever noticed it before. Then the mother began to listen to her own speech and found it was a great deal less fluent than she had thought. Both women made an effort to point out their speech breaks to the stuttering girl, who came to realize that these breaks were part of normal everyday talking and not some bizarre aberration that she suffered from. It is very important that both stutterers and their parents learn to tolerate and accept these normal disfluencies.[8]

Notice fluency. You can also help your child by pointing out the times the child is fluent. Even a severe stutterer is fluent a great deal of the time. If your child says "My name is P-P-p-p-p . . . [long pause, eyes tightly shut] Peter Smith and I go to Central Junior High," you and he will think that sentence a complete failure of fluency. The sentence had twelve words and Peter only stuttered on one. "Actually 92 percent of the sentence was fluent," you can remind him: "Ninety-two on an exam usually gets an A and is considered a very successful performance. You have been so concerned with the bad word, Peter, that you haven't heard all the successful words." Make your child aware that most of the speech is smooth and that the breakdowns are a relatively small part of the total. You might argue on this point, saying that although Peter only stuttered on 8 percent of the words in the sentence, he spent far more than 8 percent of the time it took to say the sentence on the stuttering block. That is true, but in all probability, Peter did not actually spend as much time as you or he thought on that block. Because the moment of stuttering is so emotionally loaded it seems to last forever. You might try timing (without your child's knowledge) a few stuttering blocks and you will be surprised at how little time they took. Whatever the actual length of time, it will probably be less than your child felt it to be and less than you perceived it to be.

It should be clear by now that you as the parent can help your child reduce the stuttering problem to a more manageable size.

---

8. Many controlled stutterers are intolerant of normal rhythm breaks. Some say they are afraid to let their speech stumble for fear of triggering a real stutter. The result is sometimes bizarre, almost mechanical, unnatural smoothness to the speech. Some listeners are uncomfortable listening to it.

Speech loses its paramount importance when you enlarge your child's world and activities. The myth of perfection in speech can be exploded by hearing other people's disfluencies. You and your child can change the belief that *all* speech is stuttered rather than only a portion of it.

Be open about the problem. Many parents are afraid or unwilling to use the dread word "stuttering" in front of their stuttering children. Often this is because they were advised by teachers or speech pathologists, in the early stages of development of stuttering, not to label the child as a stutterer and to ignore the breakdowns of speech flow. What was appropriate advice for the parents of a five-year-old is not so for the parents of a twelve-year-old, especially if that twelve-year-old is a confirmed stutterer and very much aware of it. It is too late to hope that the child will grow out of it at this point, and it is unrealistic to assume that such a child will be unaware of it. The seventh-grade boy confided to his speech teacher at school that he needed help because he stuttered. "Don't tell my mother, though," he continued; "she can't handle the word." Moreover, great harm was done by this conspiracy of silence over the stuttering problem. The boy was convinced that his mother was ashamed of him; stuttering must be a very shameful behavior if the word couldn't even be spoken aloud. If your child is a confirmed stutterer, be open about it. Being able to discuss it is the first step in reducing the emotional burden of stuttering. You may find that in open discussion your own emotional attitudes toward your child's speech can be reduced.

Seek professional help. Although sometimes children do grow out of their problem without any special help, many do not, and a young stutterer should get professional help. Many parents feel they are not good judges of the difference between the normally disfluent child and the stuttering child and may be hesitant about taking the child to the speech clinic for fear of creating too much speech consciousness. Nevertheless the child and you should get help. A competent speech clinician will be able to decide what the nature of that help should be.

If you have a child who has already developed a stuttering pattern with all the fears and anxieties over speaking, is it too late for parents to help? No, you still have the task of helping your child avoid a more severe stuttering pattern and developing many of the nonspeech gestures which often accompany stuttering blocks. These nonspeech gestures are often more distracting than the break in speech.

The Nonspeech Gestures

Full-fledged stutterers develop strategies to get themselves started in talking. One such strategy might be to blink the eyes. If the eye blink turns out to be a successful "starter" the child will use it the next time there is trouble getting started in speaking. The more times it is successful, the more the child will use it. After a while the starter is used so much it becomes automatic; that is, the child does it without thinking about it. The trouble is that a gesture that helps "push" the child into speaking cannot be automatic if it is to work. Such a gesture must be one that the child is aware of. So the blinking eye has lost its usefulness as a starter but is maintained because it has become a habit. The child needs a new starter and so begins grimacing on one side of the mouth to get started. For a while this new starter works as the eye blink did but then it becomes a habit too, an unconscious act, and loses its usefulness. Then a third gesture is needed, such as nodding the head. These gestures build up. It is not uncommon to see stutterers screw up their faces, pound a table with their fists, shake their heads up and down. Some children tear out their hair. There was a boy who banged the side of his head hard enough to cause worry about his injuring himself. When asked why he banged his head, he said it was to push the words out. He was right in a way, because after a savage blow, indeed the words did come out. The stutterer sometimes thinks that whatever behaviors come before fluent speech, including the stuttering block and the bizarre starting gesture, are necessary to speaking.

As a parent, if you observe some of these nonspeech gestures in your child, you can help by being accepting of the stuttering and the stuttering blocks and waiting patiently through the blocks no matter how long they seem. Even at this stage you can help by eliminating the pressure to speak perfectly. The child still feels the pressure to avoid disfluency even when the stuttering pattern has become full-fledged. Most of these patterns are self-help regimens with which the child is trying to avoid stuttering and keep speech flowing.

Avoiding Talking as Much as Possible

Sometimes children who are anxious about their speech avoid talking altogether. It becomes a great effort which embarrasses them and makes them feel inadequate. Therefore the simplest remedy is not to speak at all. They are helped by parents and teachers whose own shame and embarrassment, as well as impatience at waiting through the blocks, makes them relieved by the silence. Not talking saves everybody trouble and unhappiness. It also reinforces the children's idea that they can't talk and that they shouldn't talk. Once the child has the idea that talking is a failure best avoided, a great deal of effort and anxiety is spent on avoidance, which in turn nails home the idea that smooth talk is impossible. Your mind is really quite logical. If you believe that you can't do something, and you take great pains to avoid it and are fearful and anxious about it, it is quite true that you can't do it, and nothing counteracts that belief. If parents and teachers do their part in supporting this belief that the child cannot talk successfully by aiding and abetting the avoidance, making it easier for the child to get out of talking situations, it will be very difficult for the child to believe that success is possible. Therefore, as parents, you do not want to help your child avoid speaking situations such as oral reports in school. If your child is set apart from the others in school by being excused from having to recite in class, self-confidence is lowered even though everyone may feel relieved at the time.

Other Beliefs about the Cause of Stuttering

When you look at a full-blown stutterer it is hard to believe that this bizarre behavior could be caused just by a pattern of anxiety about talking and not by some outside cause. Many people have at one time or another believed that there must be some outside factor which causes the condition, like a microbe for a disease. Over the years there have been many ideas about the causes of stuttering, some of which people still believe. Some are so much a part of our conventional wisdom that parents who believe these causes worry unnecessarily that their child will become a stutterer.

A traumatic, frightening experience has long been thought to be the beginning cause of stuttering. A car wreck, a fire, any psychologically searing experience is thought to be dangerous to a small child as it might cause stuttering. Parents of a nonfluent child will often point to some frightening experience and say that this was the start of the stuttering and that after the incident the child's speech had never been right. My explanation of this phenomenon is that after the incident the parents first *noticed* the breaks and prolongations in their child's speech which had been there all along. Believing that a bad fright will cause stuttering, the parents have accepted the cause (the incident) and the effect (the nonfluency) and so settle comfortably on the label of stuttering which itself can be a true causative factor in stuttering. If your child has had a bad fright (and all children go through something that shakes them up at some time) don't start listening for stuttering. Your child's speech has not changed after the incident even if it does seem different to your ears. This is not to say that traumatic experiences are not harmful, but that harm is unlikely to have a permanent effect upon your child's speech. At the time of the incident your child's speech may have been disfluent (we all can lose our fluency while undergoing fear) but the child will regain fluency or whatever the before-the-incident speech rhythm was as the immediate fear wears off. In those cases of a child whose stuttering appeared to have started all at once this way, if you talk to someone outside the immediate family, you'll be reminded that the child always talked that way even before the event.

Another reason for rejecting the single sudden cause theory is that stuttering does not act like an aftereffect. An aftereffect from one incident usually becomes weaker with time unless whatever started it is repeated. Stuttering can change with time so that five years after the traumatic shock the stuttering may be far worse than it was five days after.

Parents are often cautioned never to try to change their child's hand preference because the dire result of forcing right-hand use on a leftie will be stuttering. Some years ago there were a number of studies showing the high proportion of forced handedness switching among stuttering children. There were complicated explanations that speech takes a coordinated symmetrical movement from both sides of the brain, and changing handedness would cause confusion over which side of the brain was dominant, resulting in uncoordinated or stuttered speech. The early studies had started with the stutterers and did not investigate how many children had been forced into right handedness who did not stutter. However, parents who are concerned about which hand their child uses may be the kind of parents who are apt to be worried about breaks in the child's speech rhythm and are thus more likely to be anxious that the child talk properly as well as use the proper hand. This connection between handedness switching and stuttering is believed by some pediatricians, teachers and speech clinicians. In light of recent studies on the function of the brain, I find this connection doubtful and the explanation of stuttering a little too simple. If you have encouraged your child to use the right hand when you saw there was some preference for the left, do not be anxious that you have started a stuttering pattern.

"My father and husband are stutterers. Won't my son be sure to stutter with an inheritance like that?" If you come from a family of stutterers, you will expect your child to stutter; you will be listening for it. As soon as your child speaks, every little pause, hesitation, stumble and repetition you hear will convince you that the child will have the family problem. You will be anxious to help your child overcome this affliction and will take an active part in helping with speech as best you can. You will make sure your child is conscious of speech in every way you know. Compare this parental behavior with any other parents of a stuttering child and you can see that a stuttering family is not necessary to produce the stutterer; belief that this is possible can cause the parents to set up all the conditions for establishing a stuttering pattern for their child. While you may not be able to do much about the color of eyes your child will inherit, stuttering is not inherited and you don't have to accept stuttering as inevitable even if all four of your child's grandparents are stutterers and both parents stutter. Your child may be nonfluent but has as much chance of growing out of the disfluencies as any other child. Your part is to accept these disfluencies as normal and not make your child overly conscious of them. This is especially hard to do for parents with a history of stuttering in the family who know first hand how crippling stuttering can be and are worried that their child will be handicapped in the same way. Such parents would benefit as much as their child would from consulting a speech pathologist to learn how to prevent stuttering from starting in their particular circumstances.[9]

The psychoanalytic approach to stuttering states that stuttering is a neurotic manifestation brought on by some disturbance in psychosexual development during the early formative years. In psychoanalysis the patient is able to learn just what happened during those early years and understand the particular psychodynamic in the family that led to the stuttering behavior. Speech clinicians are often impatient with psychiatrists trying to cure stuttering. On the other hand psychiatrists feel that the speech pathologists are merely treating the symptoms and not uncovering the true causes. In my opinion the dispute is more one of approach to the problem than disagreement about its nature. The two views are quite compatible. In examining the parental role in turning the normal disfluencies a child is bound to have into a true stuttering pattern, I never question *why* the parents are anxious about their child's speech or why these particular parents communicate their anxieties and other parents do not. Moreover, I do not question why some children are so susceptible to this communicated anxiety and others are not. The Freudian view of psychosexual disturbance may indeed be the basic or ultimate explanation. As a speech clinician, however, I do not feel that understanding ultimate causes is useful in breaking habits which continue on their own. Even if the stutterer could understand exactly what had happened to start the stuttering, there is still the history of struggling with stuttering speech to deal with. And there is no amount of understanding the inner self that can change history. Therefore the speech clinician is apt to say that in order to change speech it is necessary to work on the everyday speech habits which can be changed rather than dwell on the past which can't be changed. Of course if psychiatric intervention into the family situation during the formative years of the child's life were possible, stuttering and other neuroses might be preventable. As a speech pathologist I will concede to the psychiatrist that I am treating the symptoms. But I believe the symptoms *are* the disorder or at least the part of the disorder causing the most unhappiness.

9. Sorting out causes—nature versus nurture—is always difficult because in most cases a child is brought up by the same people who supplied the genes. If there were a constitutional preponderance toward disfluency (which has never been shown) it would be mediated by environmental factors.

Stuttering Gets Worse or Better in Certain Situations

Stuttering is a curious ailment. Children who stutter are often perplexed to find that sometimes they can talk fluently and at other times they can barely get a word out. No stutterer stutters all the time. Speech clinicians all have bizarre tales of stuttering patterns. There is one of the young man who stuttered in his home town but not in other towns, or the young black man who stuttered only when talking with women, the lighter the color the worse the stutter. White women didn't count and he rarely stuttered in their presence. Another man stuttered only in the presence of other men and was fluent with women.[10]

Anxiety Can Increase Stuttering

If your child stutters you have probably noticed that the speech changes with the situation and the people involved. A stutterer may be able to pray alone but not lead a prayer such as grace before the family meal. The child who stutters may be fluent with younger children but all blocked up with older children. Most stutterers report great difficulty giving oral reports at school, a situation posing the double threat of speaking before a large group and being judged by an authority, the teacher. Many adult stutterers who have their stuttering under control break down when trying to ask their boss for a raise. Most of the situations which affect a stutterer's fluency control are the same ones which cause everybody anxiety about speaking. Since the stutterer is normally anxious even in easy speaking situations, anxiety over difficult speaking situations will be devastating. Nevertheless, your child should be encouraged to participate in these tense speaking situations. If there were no stuttering problem, you would encourage your child to learn to overcome stage fright. Mastery of stage fright will be that much greater an accomplishment for your stuttering child.

10. There has been a controversy over the cause of stuttering, constitutional versus psychological or learned behavior. Even those who support a constitutional theory (some physical or neurological malfunction) admit there are psychological contributing factors. These factors explain how stuttering can improve in nonstressful situations even though the organically based condition is presumably unchanged. I feel the constitutional theory is not necessary and the psychological theory is sufficient to explain stuttering.

Admitting Stuttering Can Reduce the Anxiety and the Stuttering

One junior high boy had carefully avoided reading the Sunday school lesson for years, much to the relief of his parents and his Sunday school teachers. He just *knew* he couldn't do it. He truly believed he would freeze up and embarrass his family as well as himself. The new Sunday school teacher wouldn't let him get out of it. He was going to have the boy get up in front of the whole church and read the lesson. The boy would have been happy to leave town forever to avoid the reading. When the dreadful moment came, he got up before the whole congregation saying, "Bear with me, I stutter. Sometimes I can't get my words out." The congregation listened, but throughout the reading were unable to detect the stuttering. People who did not know him were perplexed by his opening statement. People who did know him were astonished by the smoothness of his reading. Had divine intervention suddenly cured him? Not really—he went back to his old stuttering ways soon after. By stating he was a stutterer, though, he had made his problem public. There was no need to hide. He had prepared himself for the shame and embarrassment before he had to. He knew that the congregation would be expecting him to stutter so there was no point in trying to prevent it. The contrary nature of stuttering is such that once freed from the necessity of preventing stuttering, the boy was freed from stuttering at all. As a speech clinician, I have often had the experience of a person coming to me for stuttering but speaking perfectly fluently in the clinic. I will feel frustrated because I will have no way of measuring the severity of the person's stuttering or hearing the particular stuttering pattern myself. The child or the adult will explain the sudden fluency by saying that there is no fear of talking in the clinic because speech teachers have probably heard everything anyway and expect the stuttering so there is no need to hide it.

Having a stuttering child admit the stuttering publicly is not a cure but it often does enhance fluency. The success the Sunday school reader must have felt in speaking fluently helped him feel that he could control his speech and that he could be as able as anyone else in talking. He could believe in himself.

Speaking in Unison with Others Increases Fluency

If the boy who delivered the Sunday school lesson had been allowed to read it in unison with a group of other people, he would not have needed to admit to being a stutterer beforehand to get the words out smoothly. He would have been led along by a rhythm outside himself. He would not have had the total responsibility of maintaining the speech flow. And since there is nothing physical really preventing smooth speech, the words would have come forth easily and freely. The result would have been a smooth reading even with two stutterers reading together. If your child is developing a stuttering pattern and you are afraid that anxiety and awareness are beginning, talk in unison and sing songs together. Your child's speaking problems will not be solved by talking along with someone else, but it is a way to hear that smooth speech is possible.

Speaking for Others Increases Fluency

Another surprising thing about stuttering is that a stutterer can be fluent in a play if the character portrayed is fluent. Friends of the leading lady were surprised. The stumbling shy girl who couldn't get a simple sentence out straight was transformed into an outgoing clever eloquent woman onstage. Could this be the same person? No. A good actress becomes the character she is playing. She is not being her own everyday self, but becomes another person by creating the character who temporarily "inhabits" her body. When the curtain came down, friends went backstage to congratulate the brilliant performer only to find the shy, stumbling girl she always was taking off her makeup. Your child can achieve fluency by play acting too. Play a let's pretend game. Your child acts the part of some hero and if really into the role will talk smoothly. This may convince you that your child is physically capable of free-flowing talk, but it won't do much for your child's stuttering. A person stutters in his or her own voice, personality and expression. Taking on other people's personalities and voices does not solve the problem of being able to talk for oneself.[11]

11. Some stutterers have reported being completely fluent when very angry. One man was amazed at his eloquence when his fender was smashed in a traffic accident. Other stutterers report that extreme anger paralyzes their speech all the more.

The Difference Between Fluency Devices and Stuttering Cure

Stutterers and their parents must bear in mind that there is a difference between achieving fluency for a time and a cure for stuttering. If you want your child to be fluent almost anything will work temporarily. A true cure, however, is much more difficult to achieve and in the opinion of many professionals not possible. All through history there have been "cures" for stuttering. Remember Demosthenes who put pebbles in his mouth? While his mouth was full of pebbles it was hard for him to say anything at all. But when he could manage to talk through the pebbles he was fluent. In the Middle Ages they burned the tongues of stutterers and claimed cures (modern science cannot verify them). In the nineteenth century doctors surgically sliced or split stutterers' tongues. A more humane approach was a cotton wad under the tongue. These old-time remedies probably made the stutterer fluent for a while because they made talking itself difficult, so difficult that the stutterer did not need to hold back the words. Stuttering occurs when a person holds the words back and then has to struggle to overcome the self-imposed impediment. An artificial impediment eliminates the person's psychological need to create one. Moreover, an artificial impediment is easier to overcome, probably because the person can alter the force of the self-imposed impediment.

Another stuttering treatment which has worked for a while but not turned out to be a long-term cure is hypnosis. Faith healers have also had some temporary success if the stutterer is a believer. Some years ago a researcher found that a metronome placed in the ear of a stutterer (with a device looking like a hearing aid) and set to a regular ticking sound would give the stutterer fluency. Perhaps the rhythmic ticking provided pacing. Fluency aids often produce such dramatic results that they are hailed as cures. Used alone, however, the stutterer will be disappointed to find that the stuttering returns after a while. They do, however, have great value as therapy tools. Moreover, they are valuable to give a stutterer and parents the faith that fluent speech is possible.

Long-Term Stuttering Remedies

There seem to be two main approaches to treating a stutterer: one is to train the person to speak fluently using one or another fluency aid, and the other is to teach the stutterer how to stutter in a different way which will be more acceptable.

Fluency Training

Over the years many fluency aids have been used to get the stutterer to speak fluently in a special situation and then to practice fluent speech in different and gradually more difficult speaking situations. One such method has been publicized recently as the machine that cures stuttering. The machine involved is a device to create delayed auditory feedback (DAF). If you have ever spoken through a public address system in a large space you might have experienced delayed auditory feedback. You hear your own voice while you are speaking and a split second later hear the echo of what you have just said. Most people find it difficult to talk under these conditions. You feel as if you have to fight the sound of your own voice. A stutterer, however, will be able to talk fluently under DAF. Perhaps it acts as an artificial impediment to speech and helps the stutterer the same way other artificial impediments do. The speech pathologist using this method is not surprised to hear the stutterer talk fluently. The stutterer gets practice of feeling what it is like to talk smoothly. Then the speech clinician reduces the time of delay a few hundredths of a second and the stutterer still talks fluently. Then the time is reduced still further and the stutterer maintains fluency. Gradually the delay time is cut down to zero and the stutterer is still talking fluently without DAF at all. This technique is organized in a step-by-step program under the guidance of a speech clinician. The clinician can judge how well each step is working and change the pace to fit the client. Bear in mind that in this program the fluency aid, the DAF machine, is only a tool in stuttering therapy, not the cure itself.

Another technique which can be used to train fluency is to build up the length and complexity of the utterance by gradual steps. For example, the child says one word, then adds another and then another and so forth. If a person is fluent saying three words fluently then the fourth can be added fluently. In most of the fluency-training treatment techniques, there is gradual change in speaking situation, say from talking along with the clinician to reading aloud to the clinician, then repeating after the clinician, then talking to another clinician, then to a class group etc. The successful result expected from these therapy techniques is the habit of fluency. The stutterer is freed from worrying about speech and can talk as easily as anyone else. For the school age stutterer such a technique would be very good. In the early grades this fluency training would make up for the natural fluency training nonstutterers get as they learn to speak more proficiently with fewer stumbles in their speech. It is also believed that in the early school years the emotional burden of stuttering has not been built up as much as with older stutterers. Also in the early school years it is possible that your child could outgrow stuttering even though aware of it. Fluency training would not make such a child overly speech conscious and would allow the child to forget about speech. If a former stutterer can talk smoothly without struggle or fear and without thinking about it, I would say that the stuttering had been cured.

Teaching the Stutterer "Better" Stuttering

There is a second approach to stuttering treatment which is often the best for an older child or an adult. In effect the clinician says to the stutterer, you will always stutter but you don't have to stutter in such objectionable ways. The stuttering can be controlled, the person can stutter in a better way. I feel this technique is more appropriate for the older child because it is quite self-analytical. The child is led to examine the stutter in detail and then to change it. The child is shown that there are three ways to talk, the regular way, the hard stuttering way and the easy stuttering way. The child is led to identify and to practice the easy stutter and the hard stutter (faking if necessary). Then the child learns to replace the hard stutter with the easy stutter. At first the child will have to repeat the hard-stuttered word, using the easy stutter. The next step is for the child to stop the hard stutter while it is happening and replace it with the easy stutter. The last step is for the child to learn to anticipate when the stutter will come and go into the replacement procedure *before* trying to say the word. The easy stutter will not really sound like stuttering. It may be a slightly prolonged first sound of a word or a soft repetition of the first sound of the word. Easy stuttering speech will sound fluent to strangers but the style may seem somewhat deliberate. Most children and adults find that the new easy stutter is a great improvement and are happy with their speech using it. As in fluency training there is a lot of practice necessary, especially in varied situations.

The advantage to the easy stuttering technique is that the stutterer is taught the method of self-help. Should there be a relapse, the person knows how to deal with it. The disadvantage is that the stutterer is never really cured but just knows how to live with the stuttering. For many stutterers this treatment may be more realistic.

Speech Therapy for Stuttering

Preschool: Before Your Child Is Aware of Disfluency

If you take your preschool child to a speech clinic, the child will be examined for speech and hearing. During the evaluation session the speech examiner will talk and play with your child in a relaxed and informal way in order to listen to the child's customary talk. The clinician will listen for disfluencies and will also look for the beginning of struggle and effort. Since most other aspects of speech and language will be observed, it will be possible to find out if there is some other reason for the disfluencies, such as poor vocabulary (the child pausing while searching for the proper word) or uneasiness about pronunciation. The person really receiving the treatment at this stage will be you. You will be counseled on how to react to your child's rhythm breaks and what to expect from a child who is still learning speech. You will have someone to talk to about your own anxieties over your child's speech. Even if the speech clinician does not want to see your child on a regular therapy schedule, there should be ongoing interest and follow-up with you and your child. The clinician should be willing to talk with you and answer your questions after the first visit. Sometimes a visit to a speech pathologist at this stage, in which the child is found to have normal speech, is enough to reassure the parents and prevent anxiety from building up. Some parents may need more than one visit, especially if they have become very conscious of their child's speech.

Therapy for the Child Becoming Aware of a Speech Problem

If your child reaches school age and is still disfluent and becoming aware of it, you should consider speech therapy. And if your school has a speech therapy program, your child may be helped there. School speech programs, however, are not always the best thing for the stutterer. Most of the children treated at school have pronunciation problems (see Chapter 5) and the type of therapy for clearing speech pronunciation is not appropriate for fluency. Since children at school are usually treated in groups, you should find out if your child is being grouped with other children who have fluency problems or is being seen alone. If put into a group where the sounds of speech are being taught, your child may become mouth conscious in ways that will not help smooth out speech. Of course your child may have a pronunciation problem as well as a rhythm problem, in which case the school speech therapy would be appropriate. Sometimes it is hard for parents to tell the difference between these two problems. The child would have a pronunciation problem if the individual sounds in the words were changed or left out. You could be so concerned with the rhythm of speech (how easily the words flow) that you might not pick up the fact that even when the words do finally come out they are not pronounced correctly. The speech clinician at school should be able to determine this. The main thing to watch for with a public school speech therapy program is that the therapy is specifically designed for your child's problem. Make sure that your child is not put into a speech class because the speech isn't right and that your child is not simply lumped together with all the other children whose speech isn't right. In Chapter 9 different types of therapy settings are discussed in detail.

The ideal setting for the child who stutters is the speech and hearing clinic. Sometimes there are courses for stutterers which cover a set period of time. Sometimes these courses are short and concentrated, such as all day every day for three weeks. Other courses may have two or three hours a week spread over a longer period. Whatever the arrangement, the clinic should have some follow-up after the initial course. If your child has gone through a fluency training program, the problem is not truly solved until the new fluency has been maintained for several months or a year.

If a course is not available, your child can get individual therapy at the speech clinic. Sometimes the individual therapy is accompanied by group therapy. In these groups of stutterers the children often support and help each other. By meeting other children with the same problem they do not feel so isolated and lonely. Sometimes there are parents' groups in which parents can get together and discuss the problems they share. Being able to air these problems turns out to be beneficial to both parents and children. Many times these parent groups are started by the parents themselves.

The Parents' Role

Whatever type of program you find for your child, you are still an active participant in your child's therapy. Keep up with what your child is doing in the therapy sessions. There may be certain practice procedures you can help with. For instance, if your child is learning the easy stutter, learn what it is and be supportive when your child uses it. You may be disappointed that your child is not learning to talk absolutely fluently. But bear with the minor disfluency and regard it as a great improvement over the major disfluency. Make yourself available to the speech clinician. Find out how you can help at home, both to reinforce the activities learned in therapy and to ease speech pressure, thus helping maintain the new speech. If the clinician asks you not to help with your child's speech at home for a while, follow this advice. If something needs to be changed in the school environment, talk to your child's teacher. You may find that your child is being excused from oral recitation. If the speech clinician thinks that this is harmful to your child's self-confidence in speech, enlist the teacher's help in the treatment of your child's speech problem. Sometimes teachers need a little information on particular problems in order to be effective for all the children in their class. In most cases teachers are very willing to cooperate if asked for their help.

Most important, encourage your child to try out new speech patterns in new speech situations. Remember that fluency in the clinic is only a beginning. Fluency should be remarked upon and praised. If your child can control stuttering while a preteen or a teenager, there is a better chance that stuttering will not become a lifelong condition. If a person reaches adulthood with uncontrolled stuttering, improvement and consciously controlled fluency are possible but far more difficult.

No other speech disorder is as preventable as stuttering, but it is

often very difficult to remedy. Although parents are very important in every aspect of learning how to talk, they are the most
powerful factors in their child's learning to talk fluently.

Dos and Don'ts for Parents of Disfluent Children

If your child is still unaware or unconcerned with the disfluencies:
- DO accept rhythm breaks in speech as a normal part of growing up.
- DO listen patiently while your child speaks, disfluency and all.
- DO point it out when your own speech flow catches and pass it off casually.
- DON'T interrupt your child.
- DON'T finish what your child is trying to say.
- DON'T point out your child's stutter.
- DON'T tell your child to talk better or to try harder.
- DON'T listen critically.

If your child is becoming aware or is already aware of disfluencies:
- DO listen to your child with patience and interest even if disfluent.
- DON'T tell your child to take a deep breath before talking.
- DON'T tell your child to start over.
- DON'T tell your child to think carefully before starting to talk.
- DO listen for disfluencies in others (and yourself) and point them out to your child.
- DON'T ever ridicule or tease your child for being disfluent.
- DON'T make stuttering a taboo word if your child has self-identified as a stutterer.
- DON'T put your child on the spot verbally by asking difficult questions.
- DO praise your child for accomplishments.
- DO praise your child for just being your child so that the child can feel loved for self as well as for accomplishments.
- DO understand that some days will be better than others for your child's fluency.
- DO try to relieve emotional pressures at home.
- DO try to relieve pressure for academic performance at school.
- DON'T allow your child to avoid all oral reports and recitations—talk to the teacher about this.
- DO encourage your child to rehearse anticipated speech events before entering them. For example, have the child present the report to you a couple of times before the school presentation.

9

The Speech and Hearing Clinic and Other Resources to Help Your Child

- *Referral to a Speech and Language Development Clinic*
- *Some Suggestions to Parents Before and During the First Visit to a Clinic*
- *Finding Help*
- *Public School Speech Therapy*
- *Public Versus Private Therapy*
- *Suggestions to Parents of Children Receiving Speech/ Language Treatment*

Heather was a bright, normally developing child until last year. Her mother never suspected that anything was wrong until Heather entered day care. At the first conference with the teacher Heather's mother was informed that her daughter's language output was immature for a child of four and a half. The teacher suggested that Heather be evaluated at a developmental center or speech clinic in order to determine if Heather could go to kindergarten next year. The mother was surprised because Heather had always acted bright and lively at home. Of course the last year had been difficult for the family. Heather's parents had separated and there were new living arrangements the child had to adjust to. Heather's mother had thought her daughter was taking all these changes in stride. Now she wondered if Heather was simply not bright enough for regular kindergarten.

Referral to a Speech Development and Language Clinic

The day care teacher recommended that Heather's mother take her to the local speech language and development clinic for a speech and language examination. As the appointment was being set up, the examiner at the center offered several suggestions to Heather's mother on preparing herself and Heather for the session to make it as meaningful as possible. Speech and language are voluntary activities and in order to find out what a child can or cannot do, it is necessary to have the child's cooperation.

Preparing for the Evaluation Session

Since Heather's mother had not noticed anything wrong in her daughter's language or speech behavior at home, she wanted to understand just what the day care teacher was observing that prompted her to recommend a speech examination for Heather. Therefore at her next appointment with the teacher, she took along a notebook to write down all the things the teacher had observed that made Heather's behavior different from the other children's. She asked the teacher what specific information they hoped to learn from the testing.

At home Heather's mother was careful to observe Heather more closely than usual. She wrote down samples of Heather's speech, especially in those instances in which Heather's speech was different from her own. She got out the old baby book which had the records of Heather's development. She checked with Heather's doctor on diseases the child had had and also to ask if there was anything in Heather's health history which might be significant to her language development. Heather's mother then entered the medical and developmental history in her notebook—information such as the age Heather first sat alone, first walked, first fed herself, said first word, said first sentences, etc. The speech/language examiner had suggested the notebook to Heather's mother as a way of preparing herself for the first conference on the child's communication development.

Helping the Child Prepare for the Evaluation Session

Heather's mother realized that her daughter would not show her true communication ability if she felt frightened and strange in the new situation of the speech clinic. Mother and daughter drove past the building where the speech examination would take place two times during the week before. This meant that at the time of the evaluation, at least the outside of the building would be familiar. Then the mother talked with Heather about what to expect when they visited her "special school." The conversations were not long at any one time but they talked about the upcoming visit many times during the week so that it became an ordinary and familiar topic for Heather. Heather was told she would be asked to look at some pictures, tell a story about them or tell what the pictures showed. There might be a game in which Heather would be asked to finish a story that the examiner had started.

Since Heather was to be screened for hearing, her mother wanted to prepare her for a hearing test. After the mother was reassured that the hearing test would not hurt Heather's ears, she was able to promise Heather that she would not be hurt in any way. She borrowed a set of earphones from a friend so Heather was able to become familiar with them at home. Heather was told she would have to listen for little sounds through the earphones.

Heather's mother took pains to tell her daughter what would not happen at the speech evaluation. She explained that the people at the center were not doctors, they just wanted to know how many words she knew and to hear her talk. There would be no shots, pills or medicine. Speech, language and hearing centers often look like doctors' offices to a small child. Such a look and the unfamiliar equipment can be frightening to a small child. The mother did, however, prepare her daughter for an examination of her mouth. Heather was told that since the teachers wanted to see how well she talked they had to look at the place the talk came from, her mouth, but they would only look and would not hurt her.

Heather's mother emphasized to her daughter that she would be very happy if Heather would do her best to follow the speech teacher's directions. But best of all it was going to be fun, so it was something to look forward to.

Why Examiners Want the Child to Be Prepared

Speech/language clinicians are pleased when a child has a good time at an evaluation session, but there are more serious reasons for wanting the child to be prepared for it. Most of the ,testing procedures are valid only if the child tries as hard as possible. Then it can be assumed that whatever Heather did not do on the test was not done because she *couldn't* do it not because she didn't want to do it. The examiners wanted to see the limits of Heather's communication ability, and if a negative emotional state interfered with her desire to perform she might have scored lower than her actual ability. There is always a difference between competence (the person's ultimate limit of ability) and performance (what the person actually does in the testing session). The examiners' and the parents' task is to motivate the child so that this difference can be minimized. There are unhappy stories about children who get erroneously labeled as handicapped or deficient not because they are lacking in ability but because they were not motivated to try hard or to cooperate with the testers and the testing situation. Heather, however, was primed to have a wonderful time at her special school and was going to make the most of it.

Another reason the examiners wanted Heather to have a positive attitude toward the testing session was that they wanted to see her customary language behavior. If a child is frightened or negative there will be considerably less or no language output and the examiners can learn little or nothing directly about the child's speech and language. If a parent reports that the child cannot say S and in the actual session the child says nothing at all, the speech/language clinician has no way of evaluating.

At the Evaluation Session

On the day of the speech and language evaluation, Heather and her mother finally entered the building they had already viewed from outside. After the receptionist took their names, both were shown into a little sitting room which contained several toys. Heather's mother was told to relax and play or talk to her daughter while they waited. Although her mother knew, Heather did not realize that she and her mother were being observed by a speech/

language pathologist. The clinician wanted to see what kind of language interchange was usual in Heather's everyday life. They observed how much conversation there was between Heather and her mother, how complex the language was, how well Heather seemed to understand her mother and how carefully the mother listened to Heather. Many parents want to put on their best performance in an observation session like this and try to act the way they think the speech/language examiners would approve. It is best for the child in this situation to be acting as normally as possible to give the examiner an accurate idea of customary family language communication.

After the time together, Heather and her mother were separated. The mother was interviewed by one examiner and Heather was taken into an examination room by another. Heather showed a little apprehension at leaving her mother, but her mother reminded her that they had expected this. Many times children who are not prepared for the speech and language examination refuse to be separated from their parent. In these cases, if gentle persuasion does not work, the parent can accompany the child into the examination. The testing done with the parent in the room is often questionably valid because many parents cannot refrain from prompting their child. Occasionally a child will perform in a less mature manner when the parent is present. But sometimes having the parent in the room is unavoidable, especially with children under three years old. Heather shyly took the examiner's hand and was led into the other room.

Heather's mother was interviewed. The mother was asked to describe a typical day for Heather, from getting up in the morning to going to bed.[1] The interviewer wanted to know how much Heather cared for herself, what kinds of things she liked to do, her relationships with other people, how Heather's mother disciplined her, whether Heather had problems such as nightmares or bedwetting. They talked about Heather's emotional adjustment to the divorce. Then the interviewer asked about Heather's early life— prenatal and delivery history and early developmental history. Heather's mother was glad she had brought the notebook with her so that she was able to supply all the information the examiner

1. Part of the interview with Heather's mother was structured to give scorable information for the *Vineland Social Maturity Test* by E. A. Doll, American Guidance Service Inc., Minneapolis, 1946.

asked. Then it was Heather's mother's turn to ask questions. She asked what was the expected behavior from a child like Heather. Did the divorce change what Heather's expected performance would be? What could Heather's mother do to help Heather with her speech and language?

Meanwhile, in the other examination room, Heather was playing the games she had been anticipating all week. The examiner and Heather started out by examining and playing with a few toys. What seemed to be free play to Heather was actually part of the examination. The clinician was listening carefully to her speech in spontaneous conversation. Then they played the more formal games. Heather was shown a page with four pictures while the examiner said a word. Heather was supposed to point to the picture which went best with the spoken word. At first the words were easy but they got harder and harder, and when Heather was not sure of them anymore, they stopped the game. This was a vocabulary test to see how well she understood spoken words. In the next game, Heather named some pictures in a picture book. Heather was very pleased with herself because she knew all the pictures. The examiner was not surprised she knew the words, as this was not a vocabulary test but a device to see how she pronounced her words. The words had been chosen to include a sample of every sound in English and some combinations of sound in different places (beginning, middle and end) of words. When Heather pronounced each word the examiner noted down how she had said it. There were other games: one in which Heather had to finish a sentence the examiner had started, which would go with a picture. For example: Here is a bed (picture of one bed); Here are two _____ (picture of two beds). This was a test of how well Heather used grammatic endings, in this case the plural. Heather had to listen to some words which sounded almost the same (for instance *sag* and *sack*) and tell them apart. Heather was asked to draw a picture of a man, another of a woman and a third of herself. The examiner was not so interested in Heather's artistic talent but in how many body parts she was aware of and included in her representations of people.[2]

2. The clinician was actually recording Heather's spontaneous conversation, trying to get fifty utterances (sentences or phrases), which will be scored for language complexity and maturity for Developmental Sentence Scoring (L. L. Lee and S. M. Canter, 1971). The vocabulary test was the *Peabody Picture Vocabulary Test* by L. M. Dunn (Circle Pines, MN: American Guidance Service, 1965). The speech sound production probe was

Next the examiner took a pair of earphones out of a boxlike object on the table. Heather knew all about them. There was a peg board and a box of pegs. The examiner told Heather to listen for the little *beep* and every time she heard it she was to put a peg on the board, but if she didn't hear it she was not supposed to put a peg in the board. They rehearsed the game a few times with moderately audible sounds. Then the sounds became very, very soft, sometimes so soft that Heather was not sure that she had really heard. But every time she thought she heard a sound she put a peg in her board and at the end of the test had a beautiful peg picture. This is an example of "play audiometry." The examiner wants to know how soft a sound the child can hear. Also there are different tones tested (from low pitched to high pitched). Now these pure tones are very boring and small children soon tire of listening for them. So the test has to revolve around some interesting activity or game. Sometimes the game is to drop blocks into a box or toss soft plastic balls into a bucket or slide beads on a string. The hard part of the test is to get the child to respond reliably. Some children get tired of the game and stop responding even when they hear the tone. Other times the child will respond all the time with or without the tone. Sometimes the same child will have both false negative and false positive responses. Hearing was not suspected to be a problem for Heather, so all this hearing test did was to see if there was any need for a more thorough hearing test or whether Heather's hearing was as normal as they had thought.

Heather's favorite part of the examination came last—the mouth examination. The teacher made a funny face and asked Heather to do the same, then another funny face. Heather was supposed to stick out her tongue and wiggle it back and forth. No grownup had ever asked her to do that before. She was asked to touch her nose with her tongue (she couldn't), then her ears (she couldn't do that either). She showed off her teeth and didn't mind when the examiner looked down her throat while she said *ah*. The

the *Templin-Darley Tests of Articulation* by M. C. Templin and F. L. Darley (Iowa City: University of Iowa, 1969). Heather's grammar test was the Grammatic Closure subtest of the *Illinois Test of Psycholinguistic Abilities* by J. J. McCarthy, S. A. Kirk and W. D. Kirk (Urbana, IL: University of Illinois Press: 1968). The speech sound discrimination test was the *Auditory Discrimination Test* by J. M. Wepman, 1958. The pictures Heather drew were for the *Goodenough-Harris Drawing Test* by F. L. Goodenough and D. B. Harris. It is thought to indicate general intellectual maturity. These tests would not necessarily have been the best battery of tests for Heather, but they illustrate the types of activities a child would be asked to do in an evaluation.

speech language pathologist was looking at the mobility of Heather's tongue and lips. Looking down Heather's throat while she said *ah* showed how well her soft palate closed off the back of her nose while talking. When Heather was through with the examination she wanted to come back to her special school to play. This illustrates the main reason that it is desirable for a child to enjoy the initial speech and language evaluation: if the child needs therapy, it is better if it starts off on a positive note.

What These Tests Tell About the Child

The reason it was necessary to have Heather go through all these testing procedures was that a decision had to be made whether to send Heather to regular kindergarten, put her into some kind of therapy program or place her in a special kindergarten. Most of the tests given Heather were designed to compare Heather's performance to the performance of other children Heather's age on the same test. The average performance of a large number of children of a certain age determines the normal performance for that age group. Very few children perform precisely at normal, but there is a range of performance which is considered normal for a child. If the child falls a certain amount below that expected performance, it is thought that child will need extra help and will not be able to make it in the regular school situation without it. Since the school system must make certain assumptions about children's development and readiness for learning at certain ages in order to design an educational program, the question was whether Heather's development fell within these assumptions.

Speech/language examiners ask the question a different, more clinically oriented way. Does Heather have a communication problem? If she has no problem her communication skills are normal and both the teacher and the mother need to be informed about what to expect from a child Heather's age. On the other hand, if there is a problem, they need to investigate what the nature of the problem is. That is why there were so many different types of tests given to Heather. Some tested her speech sound production, some her grammar, some vocabulary, etc. It is possible that Heather could have adequate grammar but not enough vocabulary, or good language and poor pronunciation. She may not be able to tell the difference between certain speech sounds. Very

Quail.
Walrus.
Donkey.
DEER.
Monkey.
Vulture.
Canary.
Yak.
Penguin.
Zebra.

few children perform equally well on all types of tests, but if there is one measure which is very different from the others that would point to the nature of the problem. Then if it is determined that Heather does have a problem, and the nature of the problem is known, the next question is: Can the problem be helped? And if so, how? No evaluation is complete until there is some recommendation or remediation if remediation is necessary.

Discussing the Results

A week after the initial evaluation, Heather's mother went to the center alone to discuss the results of the examination with the examiner who had interviewed her and the examiner who had worked directly with Heather. In the intervening week the people at the center had has time to score the tests and discuss Heather among themselves. The examiners showed Heather's mother the results of the tests, explaining to her what each test measured and what the results meant for Heather. Whenever the mother did not understand something she asked the professionals to explain it to her until she did. They then asked Heather's mother what she expected from Heather and how much time and commitment she was prepared to give at the present. Heather had shown some depression in certain communication areas. The examiners were not sure that this reflected a permanent disability or merely a temporary setback from the family upheaval. Heather fell into that difficult "gray" area of almost needing therapy but not quite. After much discussion the examiners and the mother came to the conclusion that it would be best to wait and have Heather reevaluated in six months. This would give her a chance to adjust to the new family situation and also give the mother a chance to adjust to a new life. If the reevaluation showed that Heather was still not developing enough to keep up with her age group they would start therapy. If, on the other hand, there was improvement during that time, Heather's mother could be reassured that Heather would make it without extra help.

Ideally the decision on whether or not to start therapy is based on the expectation of the child's family as well as the results of the standardized tests. Some families are more concerned about communication skills than others and are therefore more willing to go to the expense and trouble of scheduling their child for therapy.

Also the speech/language pathologists know that the commitment of the father or mother is important to the outcome of therapy. In a borderline case such as Heather's a conservative approach seemed the best. There are cases, however, which are not borderline, in which the child must have therapy. In those cases it is up to the speech/language pathologists to help the parents understand what is wrong and why therapy is needed, and motivate them into taking as active a role in remediation as is necessary to benefit the child. In cases where it is impossible to get as much parental participation as they want, the speech pathologists must work out a program which takes into account limited parental participation. Parental involvement is most desirable, but speech therapy is possible without it.

Some Suggestions to Parents Before and During the First Visit to a Clinic[3]

- Find out what information is necessary for the background history of your child and gather it before the first visit.
- Find out the kinds of activities your child will do and discuss them with your child beforehand.
- Observe the child yourself at home and note questions you have or problems you want to discuss.
- Present the speech center as a "school" rather than a medical facility to your small child. "School" more accurately reflects the types of activities and is less threatening.
- For an older child who is aware of communication difficulties explain the center as a place to get help in talking.
- Encourage your child to go into the examination room without you—prepare for the separation beforehand.
- Be realistic about your own ability and desire to participate in a therapy program and discuss this frankly with the speech/language clinicians.
- Ask questions any time you do not understand some point in your child's evaluation.

3. L. Cross and K. Goin, *Identifying Handicapped Children: A Guide to Casefinding, Screening, Diagnosis, Assessment and Evaluation* (New York: Walker and Company, 1977). Table on Sources of Error in Developmental Diagnosis. The suggestions for parents here are aimed at minimizing these error sources in order to get as accurate an evaluation as possible.

Finding Help

Tony at three and a half did not seem to be speaking as much or as well as the other children in the neighborhood. His speech was not as good as his sister's had been when she was three and a half. The family could not pinpoint what they felt was wrong with Tony's speech but felt that they needed help and advice. They were new in town and did not know where to go. They knew about speech pathology and specialists in communication, but they did not know how to find them. From a library search they found out about the various types of organizations which have speech/language pathologists and offer speech, language and hearing services.

Where to Find Help

The most common place for speech therapy is the public school.[4] Most school systems offer speech therapy, sometimes called speech correction, to those children in the school who need it. Tony, however, was too young to take advantage of the school services. There are also speech and hearing clinics affiliated with a university which treat communication disorders (speech, language and hearing problems). These are teaching institutions to train clinicians, and the actual therapy is often delivered by students under faculty supervision. Some might consider being treated by students a disadvantage. It is often an advantage, however, as the students bring enthusiasm and creativity to the treatment. Another advantage to the university clinic is that there is usually research going on and the staff is likely to be at the cutting edge of developments in knowledge of communication disorders and has available the widest possible range of treatment techniques for your child.

Another setting for speech/language services is the developmental center. There are special schools and clinics which deal with all types of developmental disorders, speech and language just being one area. Sometimes these developmental centers have

4. C. Van Riper, *Speech Correction: Principles and Practice* (Englewood Cliffs, NJ: Prentice-Hall, 1978). 41 percent of the 23,000 speech pathologists belonging to ASHA are employed in the public schools according to a 1976 survey. However, there are speech clinicians, teachers, correctionists, etc. in the school who are not members of ASHA—probably the majority of speech therapy delivered is in the public school setting.

full-time speech/language pathologists on the staff. Or the speech and language services are given by part-time professionals. Sometimes the children are taken to a nearby speech and hearing clinic for speech and language therapy. The public school system in many places has special schools for those children unable to attend regular classes. Speech therapy is often a regular part of the program at these special schools. Tony's parents did not think that their son needed special services like these. Other than his speech he seemed a healthy normal little boy.

Many hospitals have rehabilitation centers for outpatients. The rehabilitation centers or habilitation centers (for children with congenital disorders) are aimed at children and adults with medical problems that interfere with their ability to move around or to communicate. Often children with cerebral palsy (see Chapter 7) are treated at centers like these. Occasionally children whose only symptom is a delay in learning to speak are treated at one of these centers.

There are private speech and language clinics. Several years ago there were few such clinics. It seemed as if the profession of speech pathology was trying to discourage private practice. Maybe the old image of the "elocution teacher" had to be overcome. As the public becomes more aware of communication problems and the fact that there is remediation available, people will want to take advantage of these services and the private sector of the profession will grow. Often the private clinic for children also has remedial reading and math available.

How to Find Proper Services

Tony's parents still do not know where to look for these services. They do not know which ones are available or how they can apply for them. They need to be referred, but who will refer them?

The first resource for Tony's parents is their pediatrician or family-practice physician. They have a pediatrician for Tony and his sister, but the doctor did not notice anything amiss in Tony's speech development. However, as the doctor saw Tony only for routine checkups, there was little opportunity for the doctor to observe his speech. It is up to the parents to ask the doctor about seeking help and advice on Tony's speech. Most specialists in children's health are aware of the facilities available in the community for speech therapy. Occasionally the doctor is not educated on the subject or supportive of it and the parents have to start their quest elsewhere.

Although Tony is too young for public school, the public school system can be a source of information for Tony's parents. They can look up the local department of education in the telephone book and inquire by phone what type of speech, language and hearing services are available. Sometimes there will be a separate listing under special education. If so, that would be the place to call. If Tony's parents are lucky they will be put in touch with a school speech pathologist or speech teacher who will understand the problem and know where to go. Tony's parents are reluctant to call the school, feeling that they should not bother the school staff when their son is not even a student. They should not feel this way. The public schools are tax-supported institutions, and Tony's parents have the right to "bother" them. Moreover, the professionals at the school realize that if Tony needs help now and does not get it, it will be much harder to treat him in a few years when he does go to school.

Tony's parents could also turn to the local university or college. There may not be a speech and hearing clinic connected with the college, but if there is one at any of the colleges or universities in the general area, they will know about it. Colleges and universities usually have their academic departments listed in the phone book. If there is a listing under speech and hearing sciences or speech pathology and audiology or communication disorders or some similar title, Tony's parents should call that number. Sometimes, too, speech pathology gets tucked into a college's speech and drama department. A school of education or a department of psychology would be another possibility. If they do not have the services themselves they should know where to go to find them.

Private speech/language pathologists would be listed in the classified section of the telephone book under speech/language pathologists or speech clinicians. Tony's parents are a little reluctant to call a number in the phone book, but it can be a starting point for gathering information.

The American Speech-Language-Hearing Association has a Guide of Clinical Services which lists all accredited services available in the United States and territories. Tony's parents could write to them or call them for the pertinent information for their locality. (For the address and telephone number, see Organizations for Further Information, p. 258, which also lists the professional organizations outside the United States that could help locate speech, language and hearing clinics.)

Tony's parents could also get the help and information they need from the various organizations of parents and families concerned with children who have special problems. Local chapters of the following organizations can be located by writing or phoning the national headquarters (see pp. 258–260 for addresses and phone numbers): the Association for Children with Learning Disabilities, the Association for Retarded Citizens, the International Association of Parents of the Deaf, the National Easter Seal Society, the National Society for Autistic Children and the United Cerebral Palsy Association. There is also a directory of *National Information Sources on Handicapping Conditions and Related Services* (a U.S. Government publication). Tony's parents need not feel that their son must be autistic, retarded or have cerebral palsy for them to contact one of these organizations. They are staffed largely with parents who have gone through the same problem of needing special services for their child and not knowing where to look. They are often very well informed, understanding and supportive.

What to Look for in a Speech/Language Specialist

Tony's parents can get the name of a speech/language pathologist and perhaps a particular clinic. But how do they know whether this facility is the right place for Tony? They have heard unhappy stories about inferior training and treatment and they do not want that for their son.

The first thing to look for is the clinician's qualifications. The clinician should have a Certificate of Clinical Competence from the American Speech-Language-Hearing Association. This ensures that the certificate holder has earned a master's degree in the area of speech and hearing sciences or speech pathology and audiology and has completed three hundred contact hours of supervised clinical practicum while a student. Practicum refers to therapy delivered by a student under the guidance of a qualified clinician. Moreover, there is a Clinical Fellowship Year, comparable to an internship, which requires nine months full time as a speech pa thologist or audiologist under the supervision of a holder of the CCC. It also means that the person has passed a national examination on the specialty. Even a newly certified speech/language pathologist has a great deal of clinical experience. If the certificate is not hanging in a frame on the wall, Tony's parents should ask to see it. Many states require a state license. Speech clinicians in the school usually do not need the license, but anyone in private practice would be required by law in these states to have one. Tony's parents did not know whether their state required a license for speech/language pathologists. But they called the state health department to find out. The requirements for state licensure are usually similar to the ASHA certification requirements, but perhaps somewhat less stringent.

Finding out the academic background is only one part of evaluating a speech clinician. Tony's parents looked for a person who liked and related well to small children, somebody Tony could trust. One of the things that can make an experience with a speech pathologist a failure, even if the clinician is well educated and well trained in the field, is a lack of rapport with small children. Not only does Tony have to trust and relate to the speech clinician, but so do Tony's parents. They may have to tell the speech clinician things that they do not like to talk about and should feel secure that these revelations will be treated confidentially and in a nonjudgmental way. Parents should not have to feel put on trial by the speech professional. The speech clinician should also be willing to explain to parents in *plain English* what is going on with their child. No parent should be expected to decipher professional jargon. The speech clinician should be someone who respects parents as specialists in their own child. Sometimes clinicians downplay parents' opinions, but a good clinician uses the parents' opinions as a source of information to help understand the case.

One of the best ways to judge a clinician and a clinic is to talk to someone who has used the services before. This is why parent groups are so helpful. Often parents see things about a clinician that the clinician's professional colleagues do not. Tony's parents should not be afraid to reject a speech pathologist on "personal" grounds. If they or Tony do not like the person, and feel no strong rapport, speech therapy is not likely to do much good. Speech and language *are* very personal, and speech/language or hearing therapy is a long-term effort.

What to Expect from Speech and Language Therapy

Tony's parents finally located a speech and hearing center. The first visit went very well. Tony liked the clinician and enjoyed the activities. The parents went back to the center to plan for Tony's treatment. The speech/language pathologist said that the test findings indicated that Tony has a mild to moderate language delay. The parents asked what that meant and an explanation followed. Tony talks and comprehends other people like a child younger than his chronological age. The clinician explained the various tests which Tony had been given, how he responded to them and what the results meant. The parents were asked what they were doing, if anything, to help Tony with his speech. They were also asked if they could understand Tony's attempts to communicate and how Tony behaved when he realized that they did not understand. There had been similar questions at the initial interview, but they had been more general. Now that the clinician had seen Tony and understood the problem, the questions could be specific. The parents expressed their fears for Tony, how anxious they were to help him and even more anxious not to do the wrong thing. The parents and clinician decided to schedule Tony for therapy twice a week. Each session would be an hour long but broken into two parts—one-half hour with a group of three other children like Tony and the other half-hour of each session would be for Tony alone. At first Tony's parents did not like the idea of a group because they wanted Tony to get as much help as possible and they thought that the group would somehow dilute the therapy. The clinician explained that many children, especially those as young as Tony, progress faster in a group because the children stimulate each other.

Speech therapy for children is usually scheduled two or three times a week. If your child is in a group with other children the session can be longer than for individual therapy. Children seem to tire more quickly receiving the concentrated attention of the individual session. Preschool children do better with shorter sessions than school-age children. One-half hour of work is a lot for a child of Tony's age. So unless there is a break of some kind such as moving to a different therapy situation, one-half hour would be the best session length. School-age children can benefit from longer sessions. Occasionally there will be a child who has to travel a long distance to the clinic and gets scheduled for a two-hour session once a week. This is not the best schedule clinically. There is too much time between sessions, time to forget what was learned in the session before, and each session is too tiring. In such cases the clinician can advise the parents on little practice periods at home to reinforce the new speech.[5]

Speech therapy takes longer than you think. The most important thing for Tony's parents to realize is that speech therapy will take longer than they think. Many people believe that a few speech lessons is all that is needed to change a person's speech. For most cases this is not true. When a person is trying to change an undesirable speech habit the process often takes several months. This makes sense when you realize that many speech patterns take years to establish and if they are undesirable they have to be disestablished and new patterns learned to replace them. Tony has some difficulty acquiring speech and language in the first place and such a problem won't be "fixed" in only a few sessions.

Reinforcement at home. There may be homework or practice at home. This serves not only to help the child remember the clinic lesson but to transfer the new speech and language learned in the artificial situation of the clinic to the more natural home environment. Home reinforcement may be an everyday speech session especially set aside from other activities, a kind of mini-clinic. Or the home reinforcement may be more informal. For example the parents may be encouraged to emphasize one or more speech sounds when they speak to their child to provide extra stimulation in that sound. The parents may be asked to help in the "carryover" of the new speech patterns into regular life by setting aside some activity such as conversation at the dinner table as the "good speech" time during which the child will be encouraged to think about speech and to remember what was learned in clinic. It is a poor idea to encourage the child to speak perfectly all of the time,

---

5. J. E. Bernthal and N. W. Bankson, *Articulation Disorders* (Englewood Cliffs, NJ: Prentice-Hall, 1981). The results of experiments on the benefits of block scheduling (daily sessions for short eight-week terms) and intermittent scheduling (twice a week for longer eight-month terms) shows that for some articulation disorders the concentrated scheduling yields better results. But for the child with an organically based disorder such as cerebral palsy or cleft palate the intermittent scheduling does better. Moreover, there are stuttering therapy programs which seem to last only a few weeks (on paper) but with follow-up and a certain amount of relapse the therapy takes considerably longer.

for no one can think about how to talk all of the time.

Tony's parents are prepared to devote some of their time at home to help Tony retain what he has learned in his speech lesson. They hope they will be able to observe the therapy sessions or at least some of them so that they can understand what kinds of experiences Tony is having in the clinic, then at home they can do some of the activities together. The parents should discuss this with the clinician first and make sure they understand what the particular activities are meant to accomplish. Tony's clinic has a special observation window through which the parents can watch the therapy session without being seen by Tony. After watching a session the parents can talk to Tony about what he did in "speech school." This technique elicits conversation from Tony and helps him remember what he did in his speech therapy session.

Maintaining communication with the clinician throughout the program. Tony's parents and the clinicians at the speech and hearing center have set up an active two-way communicative relationship. Tony's parents can ask questions any time they feel the need to, and the clinician can check with the parents every time there is some change in Tony's behavior. In this way, the parents and the clinic work together to help Tony.

Regular attendance needed. If attendance is erratic, progress is slow. Too long a time between sessions often means that the child has forgotten the previous lesson and has to repeat it before something new can be started. Tony's parents are very conscientious in bringing him to the clinic regularly. There are, of course, unavoidable absences due to illness or bad weather. If your child is subject to frequent colds or flu during certain seasons or if you live in a place where weather conditions interfere with safe travel, consider scheduling speech therapy during a time you can be sure of regular attendance.

Public School Speech Therapy

Tony's parents could have waited until Tony was at school before seeking help for him. The public school system might have treated him before school age, depending on the state the family lived in and his particular disability. But Tony's parents felt that being able to have their son treated as early as possible was worth the added expense. Most school systems have speech therapy services and are obligated to give each child the compensatory education that child needs to realize full academic potential. If Tony were sure to be classified as needing special education he would be assured by law of receiving the services he needed. If, however, Tony's problem were borderline—that is, he had a problem but not severe enough to fall into the group covered by PL-94-142 (Education of the Handicapped Act)—he would not be treated. If he were classified as needing special speech and language help, he would be placed in the regular school speech therapy program. Sometimes this regular school speech therapy is precisely what is needed, but sometimes the structure of the school speech therapy program makes some problems more difficult to remedy.

PL 94-142

Since the passage of the Federal Education for All Handicapped Children Act in the United States, also known as PL 94-142, the procedure for serving schoolchildren has changed. Speech impairment is considered a handicapping condition by the federal government and by most state governments in the United States. The law states that any child between the ages of five and eighteen years has a right to whatever special education is necessary to realize that child's academic potential in the least restrictive circumstances possible. In other words, the law does not spell out the services. Thus the child's needs define the child's rights. Different states have different age ranges under this law. Often a particular disability changes the age of eligibility. For instance, in Tennessee the child with impaired hearing is eligible for special education from the age of three; eligibility for services for other handicaps does not begin until four.[6]

In most communities a child with a speech problem can be referred to a school speech pathologist for evaluation by the classroom teacher. If the speech pathologist finds that there is a problem, the child receives treatment. It is not necessary, however, to wait for the teacher to discover your child's speech problem. If *you*

6. B. C. Cutler, *Unraveling the Special Education Maze* (Champaign, IL: Research Press, 1981). The Appendix includes a chart of the ages of eligibility for special education. The youngest age of eligibility seems to be three, but in some states there are services for those younger under certain circumstances. The upper limit is usually eighteen, sometimes twenty-one, but occasionally as old as twenty-five. Usually a child is allowed to complete the school year even if the upper age limit is passed during it.

think your child has a speech problem or a hearing problem you can request that your child be seen by the speech pathologist at your child's school. If your school does not have a speech pathologist, your child has the right to be seen by the speech pathologist at the nearest school with this service. If your child goes to a private school which does not have services, it is still possible to receive these services free of charge through the public school system. Many parents of children in private or church-affiliated schools do not realize this. You will have to take the initiative and contact the special education department of your local public school system. If speech therapy is necessary your child will be scheduled for treatment in the nearest public school at the time the speech therapist is there. You will probably be responsible for the transportation.

There is a certain amount of confusion in many communities over the relationship between special education and public school speech services. This is because the implementation of PL 94-142 starting in the mid-1970s superimposed this federal mandate upon an already existing speech therapy program in many school systems. Before the federal law, children with speech problems were not necessarily considered special education children. Of course the existing special education programs did not include speech language and hearing therapy, but some speech therapy was through the regular instructional program. In some communities today all speech services must be through special education, even treatment for a mild lisp. With tightening of funding in the last few years there is reluctance to place children with "mild" speech problems in the special education population; therefore, children who would have been treated before this law came into effect are not treated now that the law has been implemented. Because there are more disabled children with more complex conditions being taught and treated at school, there might not be enough time for the "routine" speech case.

Individual Education Program (IEP)

It is very gratifying for a parent to realize that the public education system will provide everything the child needs in compensatory education. This compensatory education is not a gift but a right, and what your child is entitled to depends upon what your child needs. Your responsibility as a parent is to see that your child gets what is needed and available under the law. Sometimes you have to work at it to get your child included in the population of children entitled to special services. Once included under PL 94-142 you need to be involved actively at every step to ensure that your child can get the services needed. Built into this law is the mechanism for parent involvement called the Individualized Education Program or sometimes called the Individual Education Plan. It is usually referred to as the IEP.

Every child in special education must have an IEP prepared. Under the law the paper must be signed by the parent, and the parent is supposed to be included in the planning. The parent must be included in a planning conference to discuss the IEP before signing it. Legally the school staff cannot proceed with the plan without your signature.

What should the IEP contain? It should include the long-term educational goals for your child, the short-term goals, the methods to be used to accomplish these goals and some means of evaluating whether or not the goals have been accomplished at the end of the term. If, for example, your child had a lisp that was believed to be completely remediable, the long-term goal might be "normal speech sound production." The short-term goal would be what your child was going to accomplish during the term or school year. These short-term goals should be more specific. "Improve expressive language" is too vague to be useful. How could you evaluate it? Goals such as "correct pronunciation of F, S and TH in single words and sentences at least three-quarters of the time" will enable you to tell whether or not it has been accomplished. You should express your own needs and wants at the goal-setting stage. If, for example, you do not feel that the precise pronunciation of these sounds is as important as some other aspect of speech and language, such as "use of past tense and plurals," say so. If the goal you would like written into the IEP is unrealistic or inappropriate, the professionals should be able to explain why these goals would not be advisable for your child at this time.

See that the procedures in the IEP are implemented. The IEP includes not only goals but also procedures or means to accomplish them. You may not be able to judge the means in detail (you cannot be expected to know the clinical procedures for teaching the TH sound). But you can use some common sense. If you have agreed upon sound production remediation and some language function (past tense and plurals) as goals and the means to achieve them is a schedule of speech therapy only one half hour every week, you can and should complain, because there is not enough contact with the speech pathologist to succeed. Bring up this point at the IEP meeting. You do not have to sign the IEP until you are satisfied that your child will receive the help necessary. There is no need to be combative, but you may need to be persuasive and stubborn at times.

Sometimes school systems are caught in a budget squeeze. Special education can seem an expensive service which benefits only a few children. Your child needs your input. In fact, built into the law is the parents' involvement and advocacy to see that the law is implemented. The school might attempt to convince you that law or no law, they simply do not have the facilities to give your child the amount of therapy you think is needed. If you feel that they agree that your child could benefit from more service but they are caught by a budget which will not budge, you and they could work out a compromise. For instance, if your child can be seen by the speech pathologist only one half hour a week, and you feel that the written goals cannot be accomplished with such infrequent contact, work out an alternative. Perhaps the speech/language pathologist can train the classroom teacher or a teacher's aide to give some follow-up sessions to your child. If such a compromise is worked out it should be included in the IEP. Many parents become militant and unwilling to compromise. But you may prefer compromise to the extremes that some people have gone to in order to implement PL 94-142, which can include retaining a lawyer and going to court. You can weigh the benefits for your child against the expense and aggravation.

Sometimes professionals working with children feel threatened by parents and therefore act defensively. The defensiveness takes the form of putting the parent down, communicating an attitude of "We know best, we are the experts." But remember, you know more about your child than they do, while acknowledging their greater knowledge of speech and language disabilities. Language and speech and comprehension are complicated and subtle subjects. There is more about the field that nobody knows than what the most learned experts do know. It may help to realize that the experts are human and feel threatened by their vast ignorance of a subject they are supposed to know so much about. But don't let your own concern and participation be inhibited by this defensiveness.

Visit the speech class at school. Once the IEP is written and signed you still must keep track of what is going on. You can visit the speech class and see for yourself whether or not the methods and procedures in the IEP are being carried out. Take your copy of the paper with you and refer to it. You should be able to talk to your child's clinician or special education teacher throughout the term as questions come up and problems arise. It is helpful to phone ahead and arrange a visit in advance to set up a conference with the person treating your child. Sometimes a stranger appearing in a speech class can be disruptive without some advance preparation.

The IEP is a mechanism for your involvement in the whole special education process which includes planning, implementation and evaluation of the program. When the school year is over, ask yourself if the goals were accomplished? And if not, why not? Were the goals appropriate and realistic for your child's communication disorder? Were the methods used appropriate to achieve the goals? Were the stated methods actually used? In some cases the school people will be just as happy if you do not take an active part in your child's program. You can let them write the IEP and you can just sign it without comment or input. But in most cases the professionals at school will be pleased to have your participation. They are dedicated to helping children with special needs and know that their success is more likely with your involvement. They have been disappointed many times in their careers by uncaring and passive parents and will wait for you to take the first step toward active participation.

Public Versus Private Therapy

Sometimes parents have no choice about what kind of speech/language service they can have for their child. There are limited choices in certain localities. Some families do not have the financial means to choose. For many, however, there is a choice and a parent wants to be as informed as possible before making it.

How Public School Speech Therapy Works

The typical school speech therapy program has speech clinicians who divide their time among several schools. They spend two mornings or afternoons a week at a particular school and see the children in groups according to their ages or problems. If a child has a problem shared by many other children, the chances are good that the grouping will be appropriate. For instance, a girl with a defective S can be placed in a group with other children with defective S sounds, since this is a fairly common problem with children. Thus the therapy will be tailor-made for her problem. She will have speech therapy at the school, avoiding a trip to some other facility, and the therapy materials can in many cases be integrated into her classroom activities. There may be a boy, however, in the same school who is a severe stutterer. The school wants to give him speech therapy, and everyone agrees that he needs it, but the school clinician does not have the time to see children on an individual basis and so the boy must be placed in a group. It may happen that at his school there are no other stutterers. So the boy is either left untreated or put into the group working on S sounds, the clinician thinking there may be some way to help him in the few minutes that can be taken from the group. The help that can be delivered in this case will most likely be not enough to be much use.

Another problem encountered in the public school therapy program is whether or not your child will be selected even after having been diagnosed as needing treatment. Often there are more children who need help than there are people to give them help. So the speech clinicians face the dilemma of having to do the impossible. Some clinicians treat the most severe cases first, thinking that they need the most help, and postpone the less severe cases until later. That time may never come. The severe cases may not be finished in time to treat the mild cases. So, having only a slight problem, your child might never be selected. Other speech clinicians feel that they should treat the mild cases first, cure them and get them out of the way before they go on to the more difficult cases. They feel it is more efficient to spread their services among as many children as possible. With this decision, however, the time may never come for the severe cases. The mild cases may be cleared up, but there will be more mild cases discovered, postponing the severe cases again. I am not at all critical of the school speech clinicians. Each of these decisions is a valid decision and response to a difficult circumstance. But as the parent of a particular child you should be aware that it is possible for your child to fall through the "cracks" of the system.

Advantages of Public School Speech Treatment

- *Cost.* The public school provides services free of charge. Private therapy can cost as much as 20 to 40 dollars an hour or more. Most private clinics and clinicians have a sliding scale based upon ability to pay. Some teaching clinics have reduced rates because your child would be used to aid the instructional program. Even so, speech therapy can be expensive.
- *Convenience.* Speech therapy happens during the school day. There is no need for you to take an extra trip. If the speech is in a different place from the child's regular classes, the school often provides the transportation.
- *Integration into the rest of the educational program.* The school clinician can relate the activities in therapy to the activities in the classroom facilitating carryover from clinic to everyday life. The clinician can also get information from your child's classroom teacher which will be helpful.
- *Other special education facilities.* If your child has more problems than the one in communication, the school special education program can integrate other professional services into your child's services. The speech clinician can coordinate communication activities with other remedial activities. Moreover, the public school system in your locality may have more professional clinicians than are available outside the system.

Advantages of Private Speech Treatment

- *Earlier intervention.* You may be worried before the age your child becomes eligible for remedial services from the public system. Often the earlier treatment is started, the greater the chance of success. This is especially true of hearing-impaired children. (See Chapter 4.)
- *More direct parental participation.* You are the one who takes your child to the private clinic and so you are the one the clinician confers with. There is no teacher in the middle. You can take an active part in public therapy, but it can go on without you.

- *Borderline cases.* If your child is in the "gray" area of having a problem but one so slight that it could go untreated and probably clear up by itself, the private clinic would treat the child anyway if you really wanted it.
- *Convenience to parents.* The private clinic will try to work around your schedule and desires for treatment. The public speech therapy program must work on its timetable.
- *No worry about funding cuts.* Public service programs can face uncertain times. You can become politically active and work to see that the programs you are concerned with are adequately supported. But if your child needs services, they are needed now and will be under whatever budget system is currently in force.

There are many considerations for you to take in deciding upon the best remediation services for your child. These include your financial situation, your ability to transport your child, the time you have available, other educational or developmental problems your child might have, how severe your child's communication problem is. Also you need to decide how motivated you are or how much effort you are willing to make for your child's improved communication ability.

Suggestions to Parents of Children Receiving Speech/Language Treatment

- Get your child to the clinic on time. The time lost from a late arrival cannot be made up.
- Attend clinic regularly.
- Try to have your child rested when coming to the clinic. A tired child does not learn well.
- Schedule your child's meal so that it does not come right before therapy. A child is often sleepy right after a meal.
- Encourage your child to use the restroom before the therapy session.
- Try not to use the clinician as an authority figure who will punish or disapprove of your child. For instance, avoid saying, "If you don't behave better, I'll tell your speech teacher."
- Avoid setting up a situation of reward only for good therapy progress. Communication skill is really its own reward.
- Avoid threatening punishment or withdrawal of privileges for a poor clinic session. Keep the clinic separate from the child's discipline.
- Observe some of the sessions if possible without disturbing the therapy.

- Ask the clinician how you can help your child at home. If you get specific instructions write them down in your notebook.
- Ask the clinician to recommend books or articles which will inform you about your child's problem.
- If you have a question concerning your child's communication development, ask the clinician.
- Inform the clinician if there has been a change in your child's everyday life—change of house, illness, etc. Such events can affect therapy progress.
- Discuss the speech therapy with your child's classroom teacher. Encourage the teacher and the clinician to communicate.
- Attend the IEP meeting if your child is receiving public special education services, and take an active part in the planning.
- Confer with the school speech clinician often so that you can take an active helping part in the remediation program.

A Reading List for Parents

Ainsworth, S., and Fraser-Gress, J. *If Your Child Stutters: A Guide for Parents* (Speech Foundation of America Publication no. 11, 152 Lombardy Road, Memphis, TN 38111). Information and practical guidance for parents of disfluent children.

Apgar, V., and Beck, J. *Is My Baby All Right? A Guide to Birth Defects* (New York: Pocket Books, 1972). A brief description of various birth defects, some of which affect communication, by the inventor of the checklist for newborn babies used in most hospitals, the Apgar Scale.

Battin, R. R., and Haug, C. O. *Speech and Language Delay* (Springfield, IL: Charles E. Thomas, 1973). A specific program for parents of language-delayed children.

Bolles, E. B. *So Much to Say: How to Help Your Child Learn to Talk* (New York: St. Martin's Press, 1982). An attractive book on how children learn to talk, incorporating many modern linguistic ideas. It is weak on information on disorders of communication.

Brutten, M., Richardson, S., and Mangel, C. *Something's Wrong with My Child* (New York: Harcourt Brace Jovanovich, 1973). A good guide for parents which includes a listing of university-affiliated facilities.

Clarke, L. *Can't Read, Can't Write, Can't Talk Too Good* (New York: Penguin Books, 1973). A mother's account of her experiences with her learning-disabled child. It is encouraging because the dyslexic child overcomes the handicap and goes to college and graduate school.

Collins, N., Czuchna, G., Gill, G., O'Betts, G., Pushaw, D., and Stahl, M. *Teach Your Child to Talk—A Parent Handbook*. Part of a kit called *Teach Your Child to Talk* which includes slides, tape recordings, 16-mm color film, workshop manual and pamphlets. Cebco/ Standard Publishing Co., 104 Fifth Ave., New York, NY 10011.

Cutler, B. C. *Unraveling the Special Education Maze* (Champaign, IL: Research Press, 1981). Contains useful information on getting the services your child is entitled to under PL 94-142 but written in a militant and confrontational tone that I do not think is helpful.

Dale, D. M. *Language Development in Deaf and Partially Hearing Children* (Springfield, IL: Charles C. Thomas, 1974). Specific suggestions for parents for home training.

Denner, P. *Language Through Play* (New York: Arno Press, 1975). Games for preschool children.

Hart, J., and Jones, B. *Where's Hannah? A Handbook for Parents and Teachers of Children with Learning Disabilities* (New York: Hart Publishing Co., 1968).

Henegar, M. E., and Cornett, R. O. *Cued Speech Handbook for Parents* (Washington: Gallaudet College Press, 1971). How to use this type of visual communication.

Kozloff, M. A. *Reaching the Autistic Child, A Parent Training Program* (Champaign, IL: Research Press, 1980).

McWhirter, J. J. *The Learning Disabled Child: A School and Family Concern* (Champaign, IL: Research Press, 1977). A good guide for educational management and especially emotional needs and behavior of the LD child.

Miller, A. L., Rohman, B. F., and Thompson, F. V. *Your Child's Hearing and Speech* (Springfield, IL: Charles C. Thomas, 1974). Explanation for parents on how ear works, hearing loss, hearing tests, hearing aids and suggestions on helping hearing-impaired child.

Miller, M. *Help Your Child for Life* (Niles, IL: Argus Communications, 1978).

Molloy, J. S., and Matkin, A. *Your Developmentally Retarded Child Can Communicate* (New York: John Day, 1975). A practical guide for parents.

Montgomery County Easter Seal Treatment Center. *Language Related Activities: A Manual for Parents of Learning Disabled Preschoolers* (1973). Montgomery County Easter Seal Treatment Center, 1000 Twinbrook Pkwy, Rockville, MD 20851. Activities for parents to help their language-disabled children.

Northcott, W. H. *Curriculum Guide: Hearing Impaired Children Birth to Three Years and Their Parents* (Washington: Alexander Graham Bell Association, 1972). Auditory training and language learning in a family setting.

Osman, B. B. *Learning Disabilities: A Family Affair* (New York: Warner Books, 1980). Specific suggestions on all aspects of rearing a learning-disabled child.

Semple, J. *Hearing Impaired Preschool Child: A Book for Parents* (Springfield, IL: Charles C. Thomas, 1970). Helpful guidance on practical problems faced by parents: discipline, toilet training, care of the hearing aid, lesson plans for speech acquisition.

West, P. *Words for a Deaf Daughter* (New York: Harper & Row, 1968). A touching and poetic account of a father's experience with his brain-damaged and deaf daughter.

Wicka, D. K., and Falk, M. N. *Advice to Parents of a Cleft Palate Child* (Springfield, IL: Charles C. Thomas, 1970). General information on cleft palate for parents, including medical feeding and educational management; also suggestions for speech and language development.

Wing, L. *Autistic Children: A Guide for Parents and Professionals* (Secaucus, NJ: Citadel Press, 1980). A good general description of autism and autistic behavior.

Organizations for Further Information

Alexander Graham Bell Association for the Deaf
3417 Volta Place, Washington, DC 20007

This organization was founded in 1890 to help hearing-impaired children and their families with information and research. There is a section of the organization, International Parents Organization (IPO), made up of local parent groups.

American Speech-Language-Hearing Association (ASHA)
10801 Rockville Pike, Rockville, MD 20852   301-897-5700

ASHA is the professional organization of speech/language pathologists and audiologists. It accredits programs and certifies practitioners. Parents can obtain information on speech and hearing services available in their area as well as general information on communication disorders.

Association for Children with Learning Disabilities (ACLD)
4156 Library Road, Pittsburgh, PA 15234   412-341-1515 or
                                           412-341-8077

ACLD is a national organization of parents whose goals are to encourage research, to develop early detection, to promote public awareness, to act as advocates of LD children and their parents and to promote legislative action on behalf of the special education population. There are state and local chapters.

Association for Retarded Citizens (ARC)
2709 Avenue E East, Arlington, TX 76011 817-261-4961

ARC is an association of families of retarded persons (children and adults). The local chapters act as support groups for families. They also work for public school services for children and residential and employment programs for retarded adults. This organization is a resource for all special services.

International Association of Parents of the Deaf (IAPD)
814 Thayer Ave., Silver Spring, MD 20910 301-585-5400
This support and information organization has a special summer camp directory for hearing-impaired children as well as information on locating an interpreter.

National Easter Seal Society
2023 West Ogden Avenue, Chicago, IL 60612 312-243-8400
Easter Seal Centers around the country provide services to many people with various physical disabilities. They serve both children and adults and often have the best services for those with multiple handicaps.

United Cerebral Palsy Association Inc. (UCPA)
66 East 34th Street, New York, NY 10016 212-841-6300
UCPA should be able to provide information in habilitation and training facilities for the CP child.

National Society for Autistic Children (NSAC)
1234 Massachusetts Ave. NW, Suite 1017, Washington, DC 20005
202-783-0125
This national organization acts as a support and information association for parents and families of autistic children. They are working for greater public awareness of autism and its reclassification from an emotional disorder to a communicative disorder. At the local level there are practical services such as a babysitting directory.

John Tracy Clinic
807 West Adams Blvd., Los Angeles, CA 90007
The Tracy Clinic provides for the education of deaf and deaf/blind children. These programs can be delivered through the mail. The parent does the training following the mailed-in instructions from the clinic. The programs are available in Spanish as well as English. When local services are inconvenient or unavailable, this clinic can provide an alternative.

OUTSIDE THE UNITED STATES

Canada
Canada Speech and Hearing Association
Box 1417, Station B, Ottawa, Ontario KIP 5R4

United Kingdom
The College of Speech Therapists
47 St. Johns Wood High Street, London

Israel

Israeli Association of Communication Clinicians
6 Benjamini Street, Tel Aviv

South Africa

South African Speech and Hearing Association
PO Box 31782, Braamfontein 2017

Australia

Australian College of Speech Therapists
Post Office Box 105, Roseville
New South Wales, 2069

New Zealand

New Zealand Speech Therapist Association
Speech Therapy Clinic
44 Peterborough Street
Christchurch 1, New Zealand

Bibliography

Ainsworth, S., and Fraser-Gress, J. *If Your Child Stutters* (Memphis: Speech Foundation of America, 1977).

Bernthal, J. E., and Bankson, N. W. *Articulation Disorders* (Englewood Cliffs, NJ: Prentice-Hall, 1981).

Bloom, L., and Lahey, M. *Language Development and Language Disorders* (New York: John Wiley and Sons, 1980).

Blue, M. "Types of Utterances to Avoid When Speaking to Language-Delayed Children," *Language Speech and Hearing Services in Schools*, XII (1981): 120–123.

Boone, D. R. *Cerebral Palsy* (Indianapolis: Bobbs-Merrill Educational Publishing, 1975).

——— . *The Voice and Voice Therapy* (Englewood Cliffs, NJ: Prentice-Hall, 1971).

Carrell, J. A. *Disorders of Articulation* (Englewood Cliffs, NJ: Prentice-Hall, 1968).

Conture, E. *Stuttering* (Englewood Cliffs, NJ: Prentice-Hall, 1982).

Creech, R., and Viggiano, J. "Consumers Speak Out on the Life of Nonspeakers," *Asha,* 23, no. 8 (1981): 550–552.

Cross, L., and Goin, K., eds. *Identifying Handicapped Children: A Guide to Casefinding, Screening, Diagnosis, Assessment and Evaluation* (New York: Walker and Company, 1977).

Cutler, B. C. *Unraveling the Special Education Maze* (Champaign, IL: Research Press, 1981).

Dee, A. D. "Meeting the Needs of the Hearing Parents of Deaf Infants: A Comprehensive Education Program," *Language Speech Hearing Services in Schools*, XII, no. 1 (1981): 13–18.

Dell, C. *Treating the School-age Stutterer* (Memphis: Speech Foundation of America, 1978).

Denes, P. B., and Pinsom, E. N. *The Speech Chain* (Bell Telephone Laboratories, 1963).

Eimas, P. D., Siqueland, E., Jusczyk, P., and Vigorito, J. "Speech Perception in Infants," *Science* 171 (1971): 303–306.

Emerick, L. L. *A Casebook of Diagnosis and Evaluation in Speech Pathology and Audiology* (Englewood Cliffs, NJ: Prentice-Hall, 1981).

Fraser, M. *Self-Therapy for the Stutterer, One Approach* (Memphis: Speech Foundation of America, 1978).

———, ed. *Stuttering: Treatment of the Young Stutterer in the School* (Memphis: Speech Foundation of America, 1964).

———. *Therapy for Stutterers.* Proceedings of a conference on stuttering (Memphis: Speech Foundation of America, 1974).

Hixon, T. J., Shriberg, L. D., and Saxman, J. H., eds. *Introduction to Communication Disorders* (Englewood Cliffs, NJ: Prentice-Hall, 1980).

Hubbell, R. D. *Children's Language Disorders* (Englewood Cliffs, NJ: Prentice-Hall, 1981).

Hutchinson, B. B., Hanson, M. L., and Mecham, M. J. *Diagnostic Handbook of Speech Pathology* (New York: Williams and Wilkins Company, 1979).

Irwin, J. V. *Disorders of Articulation* (Indianapolis: Bobbs-Merrill Educational Publishing, 1975).

Johnson, W. *Stuttering and What You Can Do About It* (Minneapolis: University of Minnesota Press, 1961).

Kleffner, F. R. *Language Disorders in Children* (Indianapolis: Bobbs-Merrill Educational Publishing, 1978).

Krasner, W., and Garvey, C. J. (investigator). *Children's Play and Social Speech* (National Institute of Mental Health: U.S. Government Printing Office, 1975).

"Learning to Talk: Speech, Hearing, and Language Problems in the Preschool Child," *A Report to the Sub-Committee on Human Communication and Its Disorders, National Advisory Neurological Diseases and Stroke Council* (Washington: U.S. Government Printing Office, 1969).

Lucas, E. V. *Semantic and Pragmatic Language Disorders* (Rockville, MD: Aspen Systems Corp., 1980).

Miller, C., and Swift, K. *The Handbook of Non-Sexist Writing* (New York: Lippincott and Crowell, 1980).

Morgan, S. B. *The Unreachable Child: An Introduction to Early Childhood Autism* (Memphis: Memphis State University Press, 1981).

Mysak, E. D. *Speech Pathology and Feedback Theory* (Springfield, IL: Charles C. Thomas, 1966).

Naas, J. F., et al. "Mothers, Fathers, and Teachers as Informants on an Indirect Communicative Assessment Scale," *Language Speech and Hearing Services in Schools*, XII, no. 3 (1981): 188–191.

Osman, B. B. *Learning Disabilities: A Family Affair* (New York: Warner Books, 1979).

Piaget, J. *The Language and Thought of the Child*. Trans. by Marjorie Gabian (New York: Meridian Books, 1974).

Poole, E. "Genetic Development of Articulation of Consonant Sounds in Speech," *Elementary English Review*, 11 (1934): 159–161.

Powers, G. R. *Cleft Palate* (Indianapolis: Bobbs-Merrill Educational Publishing, 1980).

Prather, E., Hedrick, D. and Kern, C. "Articulation Development in Children Aged Two to Four Years," *Journal of Speech and Hearing Disorders*, 40 (1975): 179–191.

Prevalence of Selected Impairments in the United States 1971 (Washington: U.S. Government Printing Office, 1971).

Sander, E. "When Are Speech Sounds Learned?" *Journal of Speech and Hearing Disorders*, 37 (1972): 55–63.

Shames, G. H., and Wiig, E. *Human Communication Disorders* (Columbus: Charles E. Merrill Publishing Company, 1982).

U.S. Department of Health, Education, and Welfare, Bureau of Education of the Handicapped. *Psychology and the Handicapped Child* (Washington: U.S. Government Printing Office, 1974).

Templin, M. "Certain Language Skills in Children: Their Development and Interrelationships," Institute of Child Welfare, Monograph 26 (Minneapolis: The University of Minnesota Press, 1957).

U.S. Department of Health and Human Services. *Mainstreaming Preschools: Children with Learning Disabilities* (Washington: U.S. Government Printing Office, 1978).

Van Hattum, R. J. *Communication Disorders: An Introduction* (New York: Macmillan Publishing Company, 1980).

Van Riper, C. *Speech Correction*, 5th ed. (Englewood Cliffs, NJ: Prentice-Hall, 1972).

———. *Speech Correction*, 6th ed. (Englewood Cliffs, NJ: Prentice-Hall, 1978).

Wellman, B., Case, I., Mengart, I., and Bradbury, D. *Speech Sounds of Young Children University of Iowa Studies in Child Welfare*, 5 (1931).

Winitz, H. *From Syllable to Conversation* (Baltimore: University Park Press, 1975).

Wing, L. *Autistic Children: A Guide for Parents and Professionals* (Secaucus, NJ: The Citadel Press, 1972).

Index